The Complete Guide to Children's Allergies

BY EMILE SOMEKH, M.D.

A Parent's Guide to Children's Allergies
Allergy and Your Child
Caring for the Allergic Baby and Child

The Complete Guide to Children's Allergies

Care and Treatment of Your Allergic Child

EMILE SOMEKH, M.D.

PINNACLE BOOKS   LOS ANGELES

THE COMPLETE GUIDE TO CHILDREN'S ALLERGIES

A Pinnacle Books edition, published by special arrangement
with Corwin Books.

10 9 8 7 6 5 4 3 2 1

ISBN: 0-523-40629-0

Designed by Jerry Tillett

Printed in the United States of America

PINNACLE BOOKS, INC.
2029 Century Park East
Los Angeles, California 90067

This book is a tribute to Dr. Jerome Glaser—a gentleman, a scholar, and a father of pediatric allergy.

Contents

Foreword

The Complete Guide to Children's Allergies emphasizes, among other important elements, the fact that allergy, the leading chronic disease of infants and children, is not solely caused by a sensitivity to a particular allergen; that the heredity of the child, his age, his upbringing, and his emotions are other important factors that determine the type and the intensity of allergy in childhood.

Dr. Somekh states that allergies do not usually cause an undue scarring of a child's personality. However, he cautions rightly that the allergic child is a *child,* above all, with the anxieties, frustrations, and fears that pertain to

all children of his age; and that the additional
burden that allergy puts on his budding personality is an important factor in his emotional
balance to reckon with. Therefore, the parents
of such a child must be observant, sensitive,
and understanding of his emotional needs. It is
their thoughts, reactions, and feelings that determine how bad the child's fears become and
how his behavior will be. If a child is self-confi-
dent, he may be sick but not a mental cripple;
he will be emotionally secure, even though allergic.

Allergy cannot be cured; it can be managed,
and eight out of ten children can be treated
simply for it. But it can kill if mishandled!
And the time to treat it is when it starts during early life. Otherwise, it may lead to more
serious problems.

According to Dr. Somekh, an atopic (allergy-
prone) baby or child usually develops allergic
symptoms in a predictable fashion. In his first
year, his problems relate to foods, skin rashes,
and basic immunizations. In his second year,
his problems are upper respiratory infections.
In his third year, his home environment gives
potential allergens caused by animals and pol-
him trouble. In his fourth year, his problems
belong to the nursery and backyard with their
len. In his fifth year, his problems pertain to
traveling to and attending school, having summer vacations, and going to camp.

In this comprehensive and easily understood
book, Dr. Somekh covers, by age level, all types
of allergies a child may be subject to (eczema,

hayfever, asthma, etc.) ; he discusses all their treatments and cautions, justly, against the excessive use of drug therapy. His practical pointers on how to prepare an allergen-free room for a child, the names of camps for asthmatic children, and lists of the geographic areas in the United States that are free of ragweed pollen are excellent. And I firmly believe, after years of treating children suffering from various degrees of asthma and other allergies, that the loving care parents give a child is far more important than his atopic heredity.

VINCENT J. FONTANA
Professor of Clinical Pediatrics
   New York University, College of Medicine
Medical Director
   *New York Foundling Hospital Center
   for Parent and Child Development*
Author of *Practical Management of the
   Allergic Child*
M.D., F.A.A.P., F.A.A.A.
New York, 1979

Preface

After forty years spent in the practice of baby and child allergy, I have come to the conclusion that the average parent can easily handle the minor ailments of his allergic child if he is taught how to do so. However, I want to emphasize to parents that allergies in children:

a. Are constantly on the increase
b. Are potentially dangerous
c. Can disrupt normal family life and destroy a child's ability to study and to achieve
d. Should receive first priority in treatment, particularly if the child is part of a broken

home (in order to minimize the effect of emotions on the disease)

e. Can only be understood through a basic knowledge of immunology (resistance to disease) which is discussed briefly in the first chapter of this book

If you are a concerned parent looking for guidance in the treatment of your allergic child, you will find that the information in this book is easily understandable and helpful. Its facts are not meant to be memorized; they are rather to be looked up when needed and used as required. In the words of Charles La Russa, consider it as a thirsty man considers water when he is near a river: he quenches his thirst and leaves the rest.

—EMILE SOMEKH, M.D.

Acknowledgments

The author is indebted to Miss Josephine Dimino for her editorial assistance and to Mrs. Gloria Martinetto and Miss Karen Philiba for typing the manuscript.

The Complete Guide to Children's Allergies

1

What Is Allergy?

Millions of years ago, a child was born whose body did not understand the difference between harmless substances normally found in the environment (allergens) and agents that carried infections. As a result, the child reacted to allergens in the same way he reacted to infections—by producing antibodies (protective substances) against them. With these new antibodies, he fought the allergens in various organs of his body, causing an inflammation there. This inflammation is known as allergy. As allergic men and women got married, this weakness was compounded in their offspring. They became known as allergy-prone or atopic children.

Explanation of Terms

Atopy (or allergy proneness). This is susceptibility to a group of illnesses that develop naturally after contact with allergens. It has the following characteristics:

    a. A family history of allergy. An atopic child will not inherit a specific allergic disease. He does inherit, however, the tendency to develop a sensitivity to any allergen when he comes in contact with it. This contact cannot be avoided realistically, and it may take place months or years after birth.

    b. A reaction to an injected allergen. This may be a swelling and an itch in the skin where an allergen, to which one is sensitive, has been injected.

Sensitization. When an atopic child is exposed to an allergen, he may become sensitive to it. Sensitization can be active or passive. An example of *active* sensitization is when an allergic child develops allergy to ragweed when he is exposed to it. An example of *passive* sensitization is illustrated in the following historic experiment. Blood serum from Dr. Kustner, who was sensitive to fish, was injected into the skin of Dr. Prausnitz, who was not. A few hours later, an extract of fish was injected into the skin of Dr. Prausnitz. Within thirty minutes, an inflammation and itching developed in the skin of Dr. Prausnitz, who had never before been sensitive to fish. The skin of Dr. Prausnitz, which did not contain antibodies against fish, acquired them through a passive transfer from Dr. Kustner's blood serum, which did contain them. Passive transfer causes a local sensitivity that lasts only a short time, in contrast to active sensitivity which lasts much longer.

Sensitization can be immediate or delayed. One child may develop hayfever minutes after exposure to ragweed; this is an immediate type of sensitivity. Another child may develop poison ivy dermatitis days after exposure to poison ivy; this is the delayed type of sensitivity. The distinction between the two kinds of sensitivity is based upon the time required for an allergic reaction to develop following exposure to an allergen.

Some factors influence the type and likelihood of allergy:

    a. The route through which the allergen enters the body. Some allergens are more dangerous when given by injection and less dangerous when given by mouth. An example is penicillin.

    b. The presence of the allergen in the environment in quantity. Ragweed may cause allergies in children while they are in America because ragweed is present in abundance here; it does not cause allergies in the same children when they are in Europe because it is less abundant there.

    c. Some substances have a stronger allergenic

power than others and are therefore more likely to cause an allergy. The egg white has stronger allergenic power than the yolk.

d. The capacity of a person to acquire an allergy. Twins growing up in the same environment may develop different kinds of allergies; also, one twin may develop an allergy, while the other may never develop an allergy.

Toxicity. Toxicity is not allergy; it is the reaction of the body to a substance given to it in quantity (such as the reaction of a person who is stung by many bees). Allergy, on the other hand, may result from an injection of a very small quantity of bee venom. Therefore, one definition of allergy would be an *extreme* sensitivity to a substance which is harmless to most persons when given to them in the same amount.

Shock Organ. The organ of the body which becomes inflamed in allergy is called the shock organ. In asthma, the shock organ is the lung; in hayfever, it is the nose; in eczema, it is the skin.

What is Allergy?
Allergy is a sensitivity to allergens. These cause an allergic disease when eaten or inhaled or by direct contact.

Are There Any Dormant Illnesses
Awakened by Allergy?
There are a number of nervous ailments that become more obvious when a person has a

basic allergic constitution. These are functional disorders, behavior problems, psychoneuroses, anxiety states, depression, headaches, stomachaches, bladder and visual disturbances, low-grade fever, pallor, fatigue, circles under the eyes, and sweating. The treatment of the allergy must precede the treatment of the nervous illness.

How Many Children Develop Allergies?
The prevalence of allergy among the child population of the United States is about 50 percent, if we consider the word allergy to pertain to atopic disease, contact dermatitis, and drug sensitivity. However, statistics show that only 35 million people in this country are actively sick with hayfever, asthma, or eczema, the main diseases treated by allergists.

Is Allergy a Family Disease?
A child may be born with an allergic tendency which he inherits from his father, his mother, or both. If both parents have allergies, his chances of developing an allergy are about 70 percent; if only one of his parents is allergic, his chances are about 30 percent; and if neither one of his parents is allergic, he still has a 10 percent chance of developing an allergy. Intermarriage has made all the inhabitants of the world potential carriers of the allergy gene to some extent; anyone may develop an allergy if exposed long enough to powerful allergens beyond his tolerance level to them. This level varies from person to person,

and within the same person from time to time. It is called his "allergic threshold," and it consists of the combined effects of all the allergic reactions taking place within him at any one time. For example, a child who is slightly allergic to cantaloupe and does not have symptoms when he eats it, may have them in the presence of an animal to which he may also be slightly allergic.

Is There a Pattern to the Development of Allergies?

Although there are many exceptions to this rule, an atopic child usually develops eczema during his first year, allergic rhinitis in the second or third year, asthma and its complications later on.

Are Allergies Preventable?

1. The tendency toward allergy is lessened in a child with one nonallergic parent.

2. Allergy to a particular food item can be prevented. The following are some examples.

   a. Cow's milk: A baby must be breast fed (and not fed a formula based on cow's milk).
   b. Cereal grains: Cereals should be introduced into baby's diet one at a time (and not in a mixed form) to see which ones the baby tolerates well.
   c. Fresh juices (orange, etc.): These should be started at four months of age and one at a time.
   d. Egg: A tiny piece of hard-boiled yolk

should be tried at the age of seven months,
and, if this is tolerated well, it is to be followed by egg white.

 e. Shellfish, nuts, chocolate, and strawberries:
These foods are not to be given to the allergic baby at all.

 f. Additives: Snacks in cellophane bags should
not be used as part of a baby's diet.

The food of an atopic baby who has diarrhea
should be made very simple because sensitivity
to food is more likely to develop if the bowels
are inflamed.

Although a baby may outgrow his food allergies, it is not wise to wait for him to do so.
Food allergy in a baby should be considered
seriously and steps should be taken to avoid it.
Otherwise, the allergy persists and opens the
door to further food allergies in childhood.

3. At the age of three or four years, foods
lose their importance as allergens, and inhalants (light substances which float in the
air) become the chief cause of allergies. The
following preventive measures against these
have to be carried out *in the bedroom of the allergic child*:

 a. Filtering devices, air conditioners, and elec-
tronic precipitators have to be installed (for
brand names see the Appendix).

 b. The bedding should be made of allergy-free
material. The pillows should be made of
sponge rubber and should not contain
feathers.

c. The house must not have a damp or moldy basement.

d. The temperature of the house and that of the bedroom should always be kept at about 70°F.

e. Strong odors in general are to be avoided (in the whole house and especially in the bedroom). The odors of fresh paint, perfumes, scented flowers, mothballs, cleaning fluids, or cigarette smoke are especially dangerous.

f. Pets should not be introduced into the bedroom and preferably the house (sensitivity to feathers and to animal hair is easily acquired).

4. Besides eliminating inhalants inside the bedroom, an allergic child should avoid them outdoors.

Although it would be impossible to entirely avoid outdoor allergens short of staying at home all the time, some suggestions help to considerably reduce the chances of exposure:

a. Vacations should be planned around the child's allergies, making sure not to leave certain allergens at home while running into others in the vacation area.

b. While outdoors, the child should avoid bees and other stinging insects, grass being mowed (as this can churn up mold spores and grass pollen), ragweed shrubs (because pollen concentration rises sharply the nearer one gets to its source), the poison ivy plant, and outdoor pets (as these can be multiple allergy carriers).

Is a Change of Climate
Beneficial to Allergies?
Children with hayfever may find relief by going to areas of the country where their allergenic pollen or mold is not present. Some asthmatics, especially those whose asthma is caused by or complicated by infection, may benefit from a warm, dry climate.

Are Allergies Contagious?
Allergies are not contagious. A child cannot acquire an allergy as he catches a cold.

Are Allergies Confined to Humans?
No. Dogs, cats, and horses get hayfever, asthma, and eczema.

Are All Racial and National Groups
Similarly Allergic?
Variations in the percentage of children afflicted with allergies are mostly caused by heredity, living habits, and environment. Allergies are common in tropical Africa; uncommon in New Guinea; and rare among the Eskimos. It is almost unheard of among American Indians.

Where Should an Allergy Record Be Kept?
The Medic-Alert Foundation, Turlock, California 95310 (209) 632-2371, has a twenty-four-hour emergency telephone answering service available to all medical personnel (via a collect call) at any location in the world. Those

allergic children registered with the Foundation wear an identifying bracelet to alert doctors to the need for calling the emergency number before treating the child.

Other places in which an updated record should be kept are the files of the school nurse, the files of the family physician, and on a permanent card in the child's wallet.

Is It Dangerous To Do Nothing About an Allergy?

If untreated, hayfever may lead to asthma; nasal polyps may keep growing; eczema may spread and be complicated by secondary infection; occasional asthmatic episodes may become chronic.

Can a Child Die from an Allergy?

Allergies are seldom fatal. However, it is estimated that approximately 5,000 persons in the United States die each year from asthma because asthmatics become less resistant to infections of the respiratory system and their risk during surgical procedures increases. There are fewer than 100 deaths each year from insect stings. However, some drugs (penicillin and aspirin) and certain foods (nuts and seafood) have proven fatal on occasion.

How Are Emotions Related to Allergic Asthma?

Anxiety, fear, anger, and strong excitement may precipitate asthma attacks or make existing asthma become suddenly worse. However, the physical basis of the allergy provoking the asthma attack is always primary and real. The importance of emotions in asthma is so great at times that it may hide or blur the original allergic condition.

How Are Puberty and Pregnancy Related to Allergy?

Two corticosteroid-producing glands (the pituitary and the suprarenal) become very active during puberty and pregnancy. They cause a temporary remission in allergies (thus the belief that the child has "outgrown" his allergy).

2

Allergens
SUBSTANCES THAT CAUSE ALLERGY

Allergens are substances that cause sensitivity more frequently than others and account for about 90 percent of all the allergic disorders of childhood.

FOODS:

milk
fruits
vegetables
nuts
egg

poultry
beverages
cereals
fish and shellfish
condiments

INHALANTS (light substances easily carried by air and inhaled):

pollen—trees, grasses, weeds,
mold spores
incidentals—house dust, orris root, cottonseed, tobacco, pyrethrum, kapok, flaxseed

epidermoids—animal hair and scales from dogs, cats, horses. goats, rabbits, birds. sheep, rats and mice. roaches, silkworms

CONTACTANTS:

plastics
metals
rubber
fabrics

dyes
cosmetics
insecticides
poison ivy plant

BACTERIA AND VIRUSES

DRUGS: PENICILLEN AND ASPIRIN

NORMAL TISSUES OF THE BODY: A person may develop an allergy to some of his own tissues which are isolated from the general circulation and forced into the bloodstream through an injury or infection. Examples of such isolated tissues are the cells of the thyroid gland and the cells of the vitreous humor of the eye.

FOODS AS ALLERGENS

Knowledge about food allergy is as old as history; the ancient Egyptians, the Chinese, the Jews, and the Greeks all demonstrated an instinctive understanding of these allergies. However, allergy to food was studied scientifically for the first time only fifty years ago by Schloss who observed that: (a) a boy had

hives after eating eggs, almonds, and oatmeal;
(b) the same boy had an inflammation in his
skin when injected with extracts of those
foods; (c) the boy manifested either an immediate reaction to a food (which showed itself a
few minutes after eating it) or a delayed reaction (which showed itself hours or days after
eating it). Schloss concluded that in *immediate*
reactions to foods the allergen is the whole
food, while in *delayed* reactions it is one of the
broken down products of the food absorbed
during digestion. He advised avoidance of complicated foods which might be incompletely digested and absorbed as such by the immature
intestines of a baby.

The *symptoms* of food allergy are hives, nose
stuffiness, asthma, eczema, vomiting, diarrhea,
gas, or migraine headaches. We know through
experience that fish, shellfish, berries, nuts, and
chocolate frequently cause hives, while cereals,
milk, egg, or meat more often cause nose stuffiness and asthma.

A food allergy is usually diagnosed clinically
with a diet diary, an elimination diet, or a provocative diet. Skin testing has little value in diagnosing food allergy.

Diet Diary
A diet diary consists of a list of all the foods
normally eaten by a child in an average day
(to make the parent aware of the foods the
child has instinctively tried to avoid). If this
list does not provide clues, the parent should
keep an exact daily record of the child's diet

for fourteen days, while feeding him only food items chosen from the following list.

DAIRY PRODUCTS	FRUITS	CEREALS
( ) Milk	( ) Oranges	( ) Buckwheat
( ) Cream	( ) Bananas	( ) Wheat
( ) Margarine	( ) Strawber-	( ) Corn
( ) Ice Cream	ries	( ) Barley
( ) Cheese	( ) Lemons	( ) Rye
( ) Butter	( ) Grapefruit	( ) Rice
	( ) Peaches	
	( ) Apples	

VEGETABLES	POULTRY, FISH, EGGS, MEAT	MISCELLANEOUS
( ) Onions	( ) Beef	( ) Coffee
( ) Celery	( ) Chicken	( ) Tea
( ) Potatoes	( ) Pork	( ) Colas
( ) Peas	( ) Fish	( ) Chocolate
( ) Beans	( ) Shellfish	( ) Vanilla
( ) Tomatoes	( ) Veal	( ) Nuts
( ) Corn	( ) Lamb	( ) Spices
( ) Cabbage	( ) Eggs	( ) Garlic
( ) Lettuce		

FOURTEEN-DAY DIET DIARY

	First Day	Second Day	Third Day	Etc.
Breakfast				
Symptoms				
Medication				
Lunch				
Symptoms				

Medication _____ _____ _____ _____

Dinner _____ _____ _____ _____
Symptoms _____ _____ _____ _____
Medication _____ _____ _____ _____

If the results are still not conclusive, then elimination diets, a provocative diet, and skin tests must be tried.

Elimination Diets

There are two kinds of elimination diets. The first one eliminates for a period of one week a *single* food item in order to observe the effect of that elimination. The second one eliminates for one week *all* the highly allergenic foods. During this period, the child is fed the following hypoallergenic diet which does not contain wheat, eggs, or milk. Bread should be banana rye, potato bread, or Ry-Krisp. The only beverage should be tea with sugar. Olive oil and lamb drippings should be used as fats. The only meat should be lamb. Beets, spinach, and sweet potatoes (all thoroughly cooked with no sauces added), and apricots, cherries, peaches, and prunes (all thoroughly cooked with nothing added except sugar) should be the only vegetables and fruits.

To this diet, *one suspected food item can be added each week,* and the effect of that addition observed. If the diagnosis is still not conclusive, then the child's food intake for the next week should be limited to water, sugar, and allergy-free proteins. (Allergy-free proteins are called Amigen by Baxter, Nutramigen by Mead Johnson, Amino Acids by Stuart. Their purpose is to provide healthy nutrition on a restricted diet.) To this restricted allergy-free diet, one suspected food item can be added *every two to three days,* and the parent can observe how that addition is tolerated.

Provocative Diet

This consists of adding a large quantity of a suspected food item to the regular diet to observe the effect of that addition.

Skin Testing (*See* Chapter 3)

Pitfalls in the Diagnosis of a Food Allergy

1. In an allergy to a food, not only the *kind* of food counts, but also the amount eaten. Symptoms may occur only if the food is eaten often and in large quantities.

2. Cooking and canning alter the allergenic power of a food. (Fresh food is more allergenic than cooked or canned food.)

3. Allergy to an additive, not to the food itself, may be the cause of the symptoms.

Interesting Facts About Food Allergy

1. A food may provoke symptoms when eaten, smelled, or touched.

2. The same food may cause different degrees of illness in a person in different cir-

cumstances because its allergenic powers keep changing. A food allergy may be shed altogether if one avoids that particular food for a few months, while another food may become more allergenic because it was eaten in quantity and frequently. A frequent check on food sensitivities is advisable.

3. There is no mathematical way to diagnose a food allergy. The only proof of its existence is the appearance of symptoms when that food is eaten.

4. Hyposensitization (injections) against food allergies is rarely successful.

5. An atopic child instinctively avoids the foods that he is allergic to because they make him sick.

First Word on Milk Allergy

Some can eat their fill of cheese without any unpleasant consequences while others cannot. There must be a difference in their constitutions caused by the presence in the body of a substance which is an enemy of cheese, and this is aroused and disturbed by it.

—Hippocrates

Last Word on Milk Allergy

A baby loses his chance to live a normal life, if, in his infancy, no one does anything about his allergy to milk.

—Dr. Jerome Glaser

Allergy to Milk

In the first six months of life, vomiting, diarrhea, gas, intestinal bleeding, constipation, eczema, rhinitis, asthma, or anaphylactic shock may be symptoms of allergy to milk. The symptoms may be acute or chronic, simple or complicated with malnutrition.

It is possible to confuse allergy to milk with an allergy to the penicillin contained in the milk of cows treated with penicillin; with an allergy to the fish used to feed the cows; with a lactase enzyme deficiency (a baby's intestines may lack the enzyme that digests the sugar of milk); or with a celiac disease (an intestinal malabsorption of milk).

The incidence of allergy to cow's milk is increasing daily because breast feeding has diminished greatly in this country. Babies are now fed formulas based on evaporated cow's milk, which is inexpensive, easy to procure, and nourishing. It is an ideal food for calves; but it frequently causes allergies in atopic babies.

Cow's milk is composed of fats, sugars, and many kinds of proteins. Among the proteins, only lactalbumin is allergenic. However, because lactalbumin is different in each kind of animal species, changing cow's milk to goat's milk may ease the allergy. If this change proves unsatisfactory, then powdered cow's milk (which has been boiled and refrigerated) should be tried.

If this altered kind of milk does not provide relief, then a substitute must be found to feed the baby. This is a very important decision whose consequences must be weighed carefully; at times it might be preferable for a child to have a mild case of eczema or some nose stuffiness instead of depriving him of a nourishing food. However, if it is imperative to eliminate cow's milk from the diet of a baby, then *all* the food items which may contain milk must also be eliminated. Such foods include cheese, cream, and butter; custard, Junket, ice cream, milk pudding; batters, waffles, pancakes, cakes, cookies, and prepared flours (such as Bisquick); ordinary bread; malted milk, Ovaltine, Cocomalt, drinking chocolate, buttermilk, canned or dried milk; milk chocolate candy, chocolate creams, filled candy bars, nougat; cottage cheese and other cheeses; Cream of Rice and macaroni; foods prepared with milk, cheese, and cream, such as gravies, cream sauces, fritters, rarebits, timbales, soufflés, au gratin dishes, and omelets; Weiner schnitzel, frankfurters, and other sausages (because dried skimmed milk may be used in them as a binder); powdered milk.

. The elimination of cow's milk from the diet of a baby must be made complete by feeding him with plates and spoons of a disposable nature. Minerals, iron, and vitamins have to be added to the diet, and substitution should be made wherever possible.

Butter substitutes: Marparv, Willow Run oleomargarine, Mother's Nuspread.

Whipped cream substitute: Rich's Whipped Topping.

Cow's milk substitutes: Isomil, Mull Soy, Neo-Mull Soy, Pro-Sobee, Soyalac, etc. This kind of milk is prepared from the soya bean plant which is of vegetable origin and is usually well tolerated; however, it may sometimes cause large and frequent bowel movements, and its taste may have to be improved upon with a few drops of vanilla extract, molasses, or honey. If it is not well tolerated, feeding has to be achieved with strained lamb meat instead. The following is Row's strained lamb formula which is a complete and healthful food:

8 oz. strained lamb or 6 oz. strained beef
3½ tbsp. sesame oil or soy oil
2 tbsp. sugar
1 tsp. calcium carbonate
½ tsp. salt
1000 cc. or 4½ cups water
2 tbsp. potato flour or 2½ tbsp. tapioca flour

Combine the flour, salt, and sugar in one cup of water. Cook over low heat for ten minutes; then add the lamb (or beef), the oil, and enough water to make a volume of 4½ cups. Cook over low heat for ten to fifteen minutes. Reduce the amount of flour if you wish a thinner product.

Allergy to Egg

Egg allergy is less frequent than milk allergy, but it is a *much more dangerous form* of allergy because the touch of an egg, its smell, or the giving of vaccines made from it (such as flu, mumps, measles, and rubella) may cause allergic symptoms in an egg-sensitive child.

The dangerous part of an egg is its white albumin; the yellow yolk is not allergenic. It is important to remember that *all* egg white, whether it comes from a chicken, a duck, or a turkey, is *equally dangerous* to the egg-sensitive child.

These foods may contain eggs: soufflés, fritters, and egg noodles; cake, cookies, doughnuts, macaroons, pastries, batters (pancakes and waffles), pretzels, French toast, pie crust, muffins, meringues; ice cream, water ices, and sherbets (unless made at home from an egg-free powder) ; mayonnaise, hollandaise sauce, tartar sauce, salad dressing with egg; icing, marshmallows, nougats, fondants, chocolate creams, filled candy bars; Ovaltine, Ovomalt, and root beer; prepared flours such as Bisquick and pancake flour; sausage and meat loaf (unless ground at home with no egg) ; baking powder (except Royal and K.C.).

Allergy to Cereal Grains

Allergy to corn may appear after the child has eaten corn or corn-containing products (such as cornflakes, corn flour, corn oil, corn syrup, Karo, popcorn, fritters), has inhaled the fumes of popping corn or the steam of boiling corn on the cob, or touched starched clothing (starch is derived from corn).

The following items contain corn in small quantities: adhesives (envelopes, stamps, stickers, tapes), aspirin and other tablets, baking mixtures and powders, ices, chewing gums, soya milk, powdered sugar, some substitute egg yolks, and talcum.

Wheat can also be an allergenic food. It is used to make bread, coffee substitutes, thickeners for gravies, and crumbs for meat frying. The following food items contain wheat.

Breads: All breads (pumpernickel and rye), cakes, cookies, crackers, pretzels, pastry, pie, bread crumbs, batters (waffles and pancakes), ice cream cones, biscuits, muffins, and cereals.

Beverages: Postum, Ovaltine, malted milk, Vitavose, certain canned soups such as Campbell's chicken soup, beer, ale, gin, and whiskey.

Breakfast food: Cream of Wheat, Pablum, Grapenuts, farina, Ralston's Pep, Mead's cereal, Pettijohns, Wheaties, puffed wheat, shredded wheat, Rice Krispies, and cornflakes.

Flour: Flour and flour products such as macaroni, spaghetti, noodles, vermicelli, ravioli, and corn, wheat, and rice flours.

Sauces: Chowders, soups, and gravies.

Others: Sausages, hamburger, meat loaf (unless ground at home without wheat filler), croquettes, fish rolled in crackers, Wiener schnitzel, chili con carne, canned baked beans, matzos, ice cream, mayonnaise, puddings, and zweiback.

These are other cereals which play a minor role in allergy.

Barley: Necessary to prepare malt, beer, whiskey, breakfast foods, or fillers in sausages.

Rice: Eaten as a staple food and used in cereal meals and pastries (such as rice cakes and puddings), to prepare vitamin B, and to make Japanese sake wine. Wild rice is used as a stuffing for turkey, duck, and other fowl.

Rye: Used to make rye bread, pumpernickel bread, rye wafers, crackers, Scandinavian Knackebrod, rye whiskey, vodka, or gin.

Oats: Found in cereal mixtures, wafers, cookies, and oatmeal porridge (they can be recognized by the presence of husks).

Allergy to Fruits and Vegetables

The citrus group (oranges, lemons, grapefruit, limes, and tangerines) usually causes allergies in the nose and chest; berries (strawberries and raspberries) usually cause hives; peaches, cantaloupes, bananas, apples, grapes, pears, pineapples, cherries, and watermelon usually cause throat irritation and abdominal discomfort.

Allergy to any one of the members of the citrus group entails the removal of all the members of the group from the diet. However, allergy to the other fruits should be considered on an individual basis.

Sometimes one species of a particular fruit may cause allergies, while the other species may not; for example, the American strawberry may cause hives, while the European strawberry may not. The peels of peaches and oranges may cause allergies, while the fruit itself may not. Unripe fruit may cause allergies, while the ripe fruit may not. Cooking, canning, or freezing a fruit also alters its allergenic powers.

Vegetables rarely cause allergies and will not be considered here.

Allergy to Poultry, Meat, Fish

Chicken, duck, goose, hen, squab, and turkey should be avoided as a group in the case of allergy to any one of them. Furthermore, fowl may contain eggs in their insides which may cause egg allergy. (In order to avoid this, an egg-sensitive person should eat only capons or roosters.) Antibiotics and sex hormones which are frequently added to the food of fowl may cause allergy.

Pork, ham, and bacon may be allergenic and may be contacted unknowingly in the lard used as shortening for cakes, in the bacon drippings used to fry foods, and in the insulin used in the treatment of diabetes. Likewise, beef and veal may be contained in gelatin, in the diced veal which is used to flavor chicken salads, and in the extracts of organs of cows and calves. *Lamb and mutton are hypoallergenic meats which may substitute for pork and veal.*

Fish is a highly allergenic food. However, *canned tuna or salmon is usually better tolerated than fresh fish.* Products of the fish industry (such as caviar, glue, cod liver oil, and halibut oil) should also be avoided by the child who is allergic to fish.

Shellfish (such as crab, lobster, oyster, shrimp, scallops, mussel, abalone, clams, squid, and crayfish) are all extremely allergenic foods which should be avoided by all atopic children as a matter of principle.

An allergist does not dare test for shellfish because the patient is usually already aware of his allergy from a previous bad experience and testing for them may cause violent allergic reactions.

Beverage Allergy

Allergy to tea is uncommon; it is usually considered a safe drink.

Allergy to coffee and to its substitutes (chicory, peas, cereals, and chestnuts) is possible. Pure coffee may be found in cakes, candy, ice cream, malted milk, as a flavoring in a variety of medicines, and in many patented drinks such as Cocomalt.

Allergy to chocolate usually manifests itself as migraine headaches and abdominal pains. Cocoa butter, which derives from chocolate, is used in the making of medical suppositories.

Allergy to Condiments and Nuts

Mustard is to be found in mustard proper, in mayonnaise, in soups, in salad dressings, and in sausages. The following vegetables belong to the mustard family of plants and should be avoided if sensitivity to mustard exists: broccoli, brussels sprouts, cabbage, cauliflower, turnip, watercress, horseradish, and ordinary radish. Pepper and ginger rarely cause allergy.

Nuts are fruits consisting of a kernel enclosed in a hard shell. The common ones are coconut, pecan, chestnut, hazelnut, Brazil nut, walnut, cashew, and almond. They may cause hives and migraine headaches, and they are to be avoided by the atopic child as a matter of principle.

The peanut looks like a nut, but it is really a vegetable whose family is composed of beans, peas, lentils, and licorice. It is to be found in candy, cake, macaroons; in certain hams taken from hogs fed peanuts; in the milk of cows fed peanut meal; in peanut butter; in adulterated olive oil, cooking oil, salad oil, salad dressing; in shortening, lard compound, oleomargarine; in canned fish, canned sardines, packed olives; in some long-acting adrenalin injections.

Allergy to Food Additives

Additives are synthetic drugs which give color and flavor to food. These have practically replaced the safe natural colors and flavors used previously and their number today ranges around four thousand.

An additive should not be condemned without knowing its exact composition, function, and level of safety usage. In products produced by reputable firms, each additive serves a purpose and is carefully screened for its suitability and its safety under predictable patterns of consumption.

The symptoms that an additive may cause are hyperactivity and psychoneurotic behavior (such as headaches, hostility, slow learning, restlessness, and reduced attention span). All such symptoms have been attributed in the past to allergies, to wrong family upbringing, or to both. We know now that most of these symptoms are caused by additives contained in canned foods.

Besides psychoneurotic behavior, other allergy-similar reactions to food additives are rhinitis, nasal polyps, cough, laryngeal edema, hoarseness, and asthma; pruritis, writing on the skin, localized skin lesions, hives, angioedema; enlarged tongue, flatulence, and acid eructations; constipation; mouth chancres; pain in the joints with edema.

The treatment of symptoms caused by additives rests on psychotherapy, tranquilizers, and a diet called the salicylate-free diet. This diet was originally designed for the management of the aspirin-sensitive child. It has now been expanded to include all foods containing additives because flavors and colors which constitute 80 percent of all food additives are based on salicylates and tartrazine, which is a remote relative of aspirin.

The following are foods and products that should be avoided in the salicylate-free diet.

Foods Containing Natural Salicylates

almonds	nectarines
apples	oranges
apricots	peaches
blackberries	plums or prunes
cherries	raspberries
currants	strawberries
gooseberries	cucumbers and pickles
grapes or raisins	tomatoes

Other Sources of Salicylates

FOODS AND PRODUCTS CONTAINING ARTIFICIAL
FLAVORS AND COLORS:

ice cream
bakery goods
  (except plain bread)
oil of wintergreen
lozenges
luncheon meats
  (salami, bologna, etc.)
oleomargarine
jello
gum

toothpaste and tooth-
  powder
mouthwash
frankfurters
cake mixes
candies
cloves
mint flavors
jam or jelly
  (unflavored or
  homemade)

BEVERAGES:

cider (and cider vine-
  gars)
wine (and wine vine-
  gars)
Kool-aid (and similar
  beverages)
all soft drinks (soda
  pop)

gin (and all distilled
  drinks except vodka)
tea
beer
diet drinks and supple-
  ments

Cooking for an Allergic Baby

The meals and the recipes that follow do not contain milk, wheat, or eggs. (For other recipes, consult *Allergy Recipes,* The American Dietetic Association.)

Because commercially prepared baby foods may contain additives, sugar, starch, or salt used to enhance their texture or their taste, *it would be advisable for a mother to prepare her own baby foods.* To do that, she needs either a food mill, a strainer, or an electric blender. A food mill will puree fruits and vegetables and separate out seeds, cores, and skin as it does so.

A strainer can be used to puree soft fruits and vegetables. A good blender will puree meats, vegetables, and fruits. (Before pureeing fruit in strainer or blender, peel, core, and remove seeds.)

When the baby is old enough to eat strained solids, a mother can adapt his meals to those of the family by taking out the baby's portion after the food has been cooked (but before adding seasoning and spices) and then pureeing it.

Some easy methods for preparing baby foods are outlined here.

Fruits: Bananas need only to be mashed with a fork. All other fruits should be cut up into small pieces, steamed until soft, and pureed.

Vegetables: All vegetables should be cut into small pieces, cooked, then pureed.

Meats, poultry, and fish: These can be baked, broiled, poached, stewed, or braised, but *not fried*. They should be cooked, skinned, and deboned, cut up, and pureed. Fish (even fillet) should be carefully checked for bones before pureeing. Cooked, cut-up lamb, veal, beef, and pork can be pureed in a blender.

Other foods: Soup is a good choice. A cup for the baby should be taken out before spices are added, and, if necessary, it can be pureed.

Baby foods must be prepared with clean hands (to prevent any spread of harmful bacteria) and clean, freshly washed utensils. Unused portions must be covered and refrigerated immediately; they'll keep for three days. Spoonfuls of the prepared foods can be dropped on a foil-covered tray and then frozen; they'll keep for one month in the freezer.

Meal Planning

These are suggested menus for the three daily meals.

Breakfast: A canned fruit juice, a vegetable, a soya beverage, potato bread, banana rye bread, Ry-Krisp, rice pancakes, or waffles.

Lunch: Rooster, capon, or canned fish (but never fresh fish or shellfish), vegetables, and a beverage or a fruit (apple, plum, apricot).

Dinner: Lamb (including the liver, kidney, or glands of the animal), potatoes or green vegetables. Ry-Krisp or any of the other nonallergenic breads.

The following foods may be substituted to provide variety in the diet:

Beverages: Tea, mineral or carbonated water, or any fresh, frozen, or canned fruit juice.

Breads: Potato rye bread, banana rye bread, and Ry-Krisp.

Fats and salad dressings: Olive oil, lamb drippings, and Mazola oil (although Mazola is corn oil, it is usually permitted).

Fruits: Any frozen, dried, or canned fruit, provided the label says that nothing has been added to it besides sugar.

Meats: Beef. Commercially prepared meats, such as frankfurters, hamburgers, meat loaf, sausages, and meat patties should be avoided because they may contain milk or wheat. The school-age child should carry his own sandwich, which should be prepared at home.

Sauces: Catsup and any homemade sauce which does not contain any milk, egg, or wheat.

Soups: Vegetable soups prepared without egg, milk, or bread and thickened with rice, barley, or Ry-Krisp crumbs.

Sugars and sweets: Jam, marmalade, jelly, honey, and hard candies can be used, provided they do not contain milk, wheat, or egg.

Vegetables: Any fresh, frozen, dried, canned, or raw vegetable which is cooked with salt, water, and olive oil (or Mazola).

What To Remember While Feeding an Atopic Child

These foods are highly allergenic and should be avoided as a matter of principle: chocolate, all kinds of nuts, all shellfish, all fresh fruit in general and strawberries in particular, and corn and its derivatives.

Many foods are related to one another because they belong to the same family, and allergy to one member of the family often means allergy to the other members. Examples of foods belonging to the same family are listed below.

Apple: Pear, quince
Chocolate: Cocoa, cola drinks
Citrus fruits: Orange, lemon, grapefruit, lime, tangerine, kumquat, citron
Ginger: Cardamom, tumeric

Cereal: Wheat, corn, rice, oats, barley, rye
Melon: Watermelon, cucumber, cantaloupe, pumpkin, squash
Mustard: Turnip, radish, horseradish, watercress, cabbage, broccoli, brussels sprouts, cauliflower
Onion: Garlic, asparagus, chives
Parsley: Carrot, celery
Pea: Peanut, beans
Plum: Cherry, peach, apricot, nectarine, almond
Potato: Tomato, eggplant, pepper
Berry: Strawberry, raspberry, blackberry
Walnut: Pecan, butternut
Fowl: Chicken, duck, goose, pigeon, quail, pheasant

Mistakes are easily made because although the following foods look alike, they are not related to each other.

White potato and sweet potato
Grapes, plums, and apples
Coffee, tea, and chocolate
Fish and shellfish

Conversely, these foods are really related to one another but do not look alike.

Apple and pear
Peach and plum
Pea, bean, and peanut
Wheat, corn, barley, and rice
Cucumber and melon
Carrot and celery

Recipes

There can never be enough recipes to help a frustrated mother please her hungry child if he suffers from mutiple food allergies. The following recipes provide some variety in a hypoallergenic daily menu. However, if the child is allergic to one of the foods listed, the recipe that contains that food should not be used.

Herb Krisps

| 13 Ry-Krisp (1 pack) | ½ tsp. basil, thyme, |
| 2 tbsp. shortening | ginger, *or* celery salt |

Heat oven to 350°F. Spread crackers lightly with herb spread. Place on rack in a shallow pan. Toast for 5 minutes. Serve warm or cold.

Cinnamon Krisps

| 13 Ry-Krisp (1 pack) | 2 tbsp. sugar |
| 2 tbsp. shortening | 1 tbsp. cinnamon |

Heat oven to hot (400°F) Spread crackers with shortening. Sprinkle with sugar-cinnamon mixture. Bake 5 minutes. Serve warm or cold.

Toasted Ry-Krisp

Put Ry-Krisp in a 350°F oven for 5 minutes. This restores oven crispness and increases the delicious rye flavor.

Meat And Poultry Stuffing

24 Ry-Krisp crackers	2 tbsp. finely cut onion
¾ cup hot meat stock	½ tsp. poultry seasoning
¼ cup shortening	¼ tsp. salt
¼ cup finely cut celery	2 tbsp. finely cut parsley
⅛ tsp. pepper	2 tbsp. finely cut green pepper

Break Ry-Krisp into small pieces. Soak in hot stock. Add remaining ingredients. Mix well. Plan on approximately 1 cup per pound of bird. Place in greased casserole and bake for 30 minutes, or until brown, in a moderately warm oven (325°F). Yields 3 cups.

Ry-Krisp Crumb Crust

15 Ry-Krisp crackers	⅓ cup melted shortening
¼ cup sugar	2 tsp. hot water

Grease an 8-inch pie plate. Roll Ry-Krisp fine enough to make 1 cup of crumbs. Combine crumbs and sugar. Add the shortening and water. Blend thoroughly. Press crumbs carefully, evenly, and firmly onto the bottom and sides of pie plate. Form an edge around the top of the crust, but not on the rim of the plate. Chill thoroughly. Fill with a fruit or gelatin filling. Place the pie plate in hot water for a minute before cutting.

Rice Pancakes

1 cup cooked rice	2 eggs, slightly beaten
¼ tsp. salt	2 tbsp. minced green onions

⅛ tsp. pepper
soy sauce
2 tbsp. corn-
    free oil
2 tbsp. minced green celery
2 tbsp. minced water chestnuts

Combine rice, onions, celery, water chestnuts, eggs, salt, and pepper. Heat oil in skillet, add rice and egg mixture, and spread gently to cover bottom of pan. Cook over low heat until the eggs are set. Loosen carefully with a spatula and place on a hot serving plate. Serve with soy sauce (see recipe below). Serves four.

Soy Sauce

1½ cups water
1½ tbsp. cornstarch
1 tbsp. soy sauce
3 bouillon cubes

Blend water and cornstarch. Add soy sauce and bouillon cubes and cook over low heat, stirring constantly until mixture is thickened and translucent. Makes about 1½ cups.

Soyalac Waffles

1 cup Soyalac (concentrated liquid)
1 cup flour (use any flour allowed
    on your list)
1 tbsp. oil
½ tsp. salt
1 tbsp. brown sugar

Mix thoroughly and bake in hot waffle iron until nicely brown. These waffles are raised by steam and take a few minutes longer than the other type of waffle. You must use a heavy waffle iron for success with this recipe.

Variations:

Use all cornmeal or corn flour.
Use ¾ cup cornmeal and ¼ cup soy flour.
Use all rye, all buckwheat, or all oatmeal.
Use any combination of flour equaling 1 cup.

Soyalac Fruit Drink

½ cup Soyalac
½ cup finely crushed ice
½ cup apricot juice or nectar
Liquefy and serve at once.

Note: 1 tbsp. orange or lemon juice, if permitted, would add another variety to this drink. Yields approximately 1½ cups.

Soyalac Tropical Drink

½ cup Soyalac (liquid)
½ cup pineapple juice
1 tbsp. berry concentrate (Loma Linda, boysenberry punch, or other berry punches)
½ cup banana
½ cup water
Combine ingredients and liquefy totally. Banana may be mashed and whipped into the other ingredients. Chill and serve.

Creamed Fresh Pea Soup

½ cup Soyalac (liquid)
½ cup water
1 package uncooked frozen peas
(slightly thawed)
Blend together until very smooth. Add ¼ to ½ cup extra water if too thick. Salt to taste and

heat. Serve at once. Any other frozen vegetable may be used in place of peas, *except corn*.

Variation: Using basic cream sauce recipe for cream soup, use 1 cup of thin cream sauce plus ½ cup finely chopped or pureed vegetables. Season to taste.

Tomato Cream Soup

   1¼ cups condensed tomato soup
   ⅔ cup Mull-Soy
   ⅔ cup water

Blend together all ingredients in a saucepan. Cook over low heat to serving temperature. Serve at once. Makes 2½ cups.

Note: Canned condensed soups not containing milk or strained vegetables may be used in place of the condensed tomato soup.

Lentil Meat Loaf

---

   1 pound ground meat
   ⅔ cup Soyalac (liquid)
   1 tsp. salt
   1 cup cooked rice
   2 cups cooked lentils, mashed
   ½ cup choppel celery
   ½ tsp. sage
   ⅔ cup water

Mix thoroughly and bake in greased casserole for 45 minutes at 350°F. Serve with tomato gravy.

Meat-Rice Patties

½ pound ground beef
¾ cup cooked rice
½ to ¾ tsp. salt
¼ cup Mull-Soy

Combine all ingredients. Shape into patties, using ¼ cup mixture for each patty. Place on broiler pan, 3 inches from heat, and cook until browned on both sides. Serve hot. Makes 6 patties.

Baked Chicken

4- to 5-pound hen
potato flour
salt
pepper
chicken fat
onion
water

Cut chicken into serving pieces. Roll in flour seasoned with salt and pepper and brown in frying pan. Remove to roaster. Chop onion into small pieces, add to water, and add chicken.

Eggplant and Tomatoes

---

3 slices of bacon, chopped fine
2 cups fresh tomatoes, peeled
    and diced
salt
2 cups uncooked eggplant, diced
½ cup onions, chopped fine
pepper

Fry bacon, then add onions and cook until they are transparent. Then add the eggplant. Cook about 15 to 20 minutes over low heat and add the fresh tomatoes and seasoning. Serves four.

Baked Sweet Potatoes

Serve 1 baked sweet potato with 1 tsp. chicken fat.

Baked White Potatoes

Serve 1 baked potato with 1 tsp. chicken fat.

Butter Bits

- ½ cup arrowroot
- 1 cup soft corn-free margarine
- 1 cup sifted potato or rice flour
- ½ cup cane or beet confectioner's sugar

Mix and sift flour, arrowroot, and sugar. Blend margarine into flour mixture with wooden spoon to make a soft dough. Shape into a ball and wrap in waxed paper. Chill well. Shape dough into 1-inch balls. Place on ungreased baking sheets about 2 inches apart. Flatten with lightly floured fork. Bake 20 minutes at 300°F. Makes about two dozen bits.

Apricot Rice Pudding

- 1 tbsp. uncooked rice
- ¾ cup hot water
- ¼ cup Mull-Soy
- pinch salt
- 2 tbsp. cane or beet brown sugar
- ¼ cup strained, stewed apricots
- ¼ tsp. vanilla

Mash rice and put in 1-pint baking dish. Add water, Mull-Soy, salt, and sugar and blend well. Bake in moderately warm oven (325°F) for 1½ hours, stirring occasionally. Remove from oven and stir in strained apricots and vanilla. Return to oven and continue baking for ½ hour longer. Cool at room temperature and then chill in refrigerator. Serve cold.

Banana Rye Bread

---

   2 packages cake yeast
   1 tbsp. salt
   ¼ cup warm (not hot) water
   1½ tbsp. sugar
   3 tbsp. vegetable shortening, melted, or 3 tbsp.
      vegetable oil
   2½ cups mashed ripe bananas
      (5 to 6 bananas)*
   5½ to 6 cups rye flour

Dissolve yeast in water. In large bowl, mix together salt, sugar, shortening, and bananas. Add three cups of flour and beat until smooth. Beat in the dissolved yeast. Add 2½ cups flour gradually and mix well.

   Place dough on floured board, adding just enough additional rye flour to prevent sticking (about 6 tbsp.). Knead lightly for about 4 minutes. Place dough into lightly greased bowl. Cover bowl. Let rise in warm place until double in bulk (about 2 hours). Place dough again on floured board (2 to 3 tbsp. flour) and knead lightly about 2 minutes.

*Use fully ripe bananas (yellow peel flecked with brown).

Grease bottoms only of 2 bread pans (3 x 4 x 3 inches). Shape dough into 2 loaves, place in pans, and cover. Let dough rise again in a warm place until loaves double in bulk (about 1 hour).

Bake in a hot oven (425°F) 5 to 10 minutes, or until crust begins to brown. Reduce temperature to 350°F and bake 35 to 40 minutes longer, or until bread is done.*

Remove from oven. Brush top crust with shortening. Remove from pans. Makes 2 loaves.

Dough may be shaped into rolls and baked in muffin pans or on sheet pans (grease bottoms only). Bake at 350°F for 20 to 25 minutes, depending on size of roll. Remove from oven and proceed as with bread. For variety, sprinkle caraway seeds on top of dough before baking.

All measurements used in this recipe are level.

INHALANTS AS ALLERGENS

Inhalants are allergens which are light enough to float in the air. The main ones are pollen, molds, incidentals, and epidermoids.

Pollen is the most potent inhalant. It is a yellow powder which acts as the male fertilizing agent of a flower.

Insect-transported pollen rarely causes allergies; rather, allergies are caused by wind-disseminated pollen originating in small flowers

*Tests for completely baked bread: golden brown crust on top and bottom, loaf has hollow sound when tapped, loaf shrinks slightly from the pan side.

which have no nectar or scent. This type of pollen pollutes the air of an inhabited area because it is produced in quantity, is light enough to be easily transported by wind, and has allergenic powers. Such pollen falls into three categories:

    a. Pollen that has little allergenic power but is produced in abundance, like the pollen of the pine tree.

    b. Pollen that has great allergenic power but is produced in small quantities, like the pollen of the Russian thistle.

    c. Pollen that has great allergenic power and is produced in large quantities, like the pollen of the ragweed plant. This pollen is the main cause of allergy in the United States. (High humidity and cold weather diminish its allergenic powers.)

Allergenic pollen may be produced by trees, grasses, and weeds.

Characteristics of the Trees
That Cause Pollen Allergy

The following trees pollinate in the United States about the end of April and their pollination lasts from two to three weeks: oak, poplar, beech, elm, hickory, ash, birch, and maple. They can be recognized by their shape, bark, flowers, fruits, and leaves.

The oak is a stout and tall tree that grows to a height of from 60 to 100 feet; it has a leaf with deep, rounded lobes; and it changes its color with the seasons.

The poplar is a tree found on river banks; it grows to a height of up to 100 feet; its leaf is very broad in relation to its length.

The beech has the smoothest bark of all trees. It produces nuts with prickly husks that crack open; leaves that have neat, straight veins; and roots that are flat and large, with moss around them.

The elm is stout and spreads its branches like an umbrella.

The shagback hickory has the shaggiest bark of all trees; it produces very tasty nuts; its wood is strong and tough.

The ash grows up to twenty-five feet tall on slopes and near swamps; its flowers grow in thick clusters.

The white birch shines best in moonlight while the other trees look dark. It is called canoe birch because the Indians peeled its bark to make canoes. It grows in sunny places.

The maple has a sugary sap; its seeds have wings that hang in pairs.

Characteristics of the Grasses That Cause Allergy

Grasses cause three times as many allergies as trees because they grow almost anywhere in the world (from the frozen North to the equator), even though they thrive best in moderate climates. There are many kinds of grasses, some of which, like sugar cane, wheat, rye, corn, bamboo, and rice, are planted so far from human habitations that they rarely cause allergies. Timothy, Johnson orchard, Bermuda, blue, and June are the names of grasses which can cause allergies. They grow in meadows and lawns in and around densely populated areas and pollinate in the United States from May to August.

Allergy to grasses is easily diagnosed because the pollen of all grasses looks the same when seen under a microscope; as a result, the pollen of any kind of grass can be used for testing or desensitization. (There are two exceptions to this rule: Bermuda and Johnson grasses, which have importance only in limited localities.)

In subtropical countries like Israel, grasses pollinate all year around and are the main cause of pollen allergy.

Characteristics of the Weeds
That Cause Allergies

The most common cause of pollen allergy in the United States is weeds.

Some weeds, like English plantain, pollinate in June and July, while ragweed pollinates from the middle of August to the first frost. There is a short variety of ragweed, a tall variety, and a giant one. The short variety reaches a height of one to five feet and has hairy green stems, parted leaves, and long green-to-yellow spikes. The giant variety may reach a height of fifteen feet and has either three-lobed or simple leaves.

Both plants can live in the poorest of soils and can resist all severe weather conditions but snow. About mid-August, a photochemical reaction (which depends upon the balance between daylight and darkness) causes all ragweed plants to produce flower spikes which contain pollen. After a day or two, pressure builds up in the spikes, they burst open, and the pollen is thrown out into the air. It lands on the plant's leaves, dries up, and is then carried away by the wind for hundreds of miles. All ragweed pollen looks and acts very much alike, no matter what variety of ragweed plant originated it.

For the seasons of pollination of trees, grasses, and weeds, see the Appendix.

Molds

Molds are very small plants which nature uses as scavengers of the soil to convert dead leaves into fertilizer. They have no roots, stems, leaves, or chlorophyll, and they live as parasites because they nourish themselves from dead leaves, old shoes, walls of damp basements, old paper—almost anything except metal.

The mold plant is composed of threads that intertwine into a loose network on which grow the fruits of the plant, or its spores. When a spore lands on good soil, it sends some threads into the ground to form roots, while other threads grow upward and form a sort of a tree.

Molds live best at a temperature of 70° to 90°F; they stop growing at 40°F. They are killed by high temperatures, but survive freezing for months.

Mold spores leave their mother-dwelling during the summer months and are scattered by winds and storms for miles around their locality. Each locality has its own brand of molds. It takes a special mold survey to determine the type of molds found in a particular place. This is done by exposing a plate, which contains mold food, to the open air for a number of minutes each day.

Here are the results of a survey made by Center Laboratories for the Port Washington area on Long Island, New York, regarding four common molds:

Alternaria. Out of 100 mold colonies grown in a culture plate, 80 contained alternaria (i.e., 80 percent). This is a mold which looks dirty gray and is found in decaying vegetation.

Hormodendrum. Seventy-six percent. This mold on culture looks similar to alternaria. It is likewise found in decaying vegetation, as well as on dead tobacco leaves, tomatoes, or peaches.

Penicillium. Sixty-seven percent. This mold looks blue on culture. It is the common bread mold, as well as the factor in the ripening of the Camembert and Roquefort cheeses.

Aspergillus. Twenty-four percent. This is a black mold found on the walls of old, damp, and musty houses.

The chapter in our medical textbooks on mold allergy is a relatively new one. It was added in 1923 when Van Leuwen of Holland (a country full of damp canals) described cases of asthma caused by molds. He was followed in

1924 by Jimenes Diaz of Spain, who studied the climatic and coastal asthma of Barcelona which he ascribed to molds. These two allergists were followed in 1930 by Durham and Feinberg, who studied mold asthma extensively in America. In 1952, for the first time in the history of the Middle East, I exposed plates, cultured molds, and desensitized against them in Tel Aviv.

Mold allergy is a disorder which is similar in character to pollen allergy because molds do not have to attach themselves to an organ of the body to cause disease (fungi in feet cause disease, but not allergies) ; they simply have to be present in the air to do so.

Today there is a world increase in the number of people who are suffering from mold allergy. This is caused by two factors:

    a. The discovery of oil in the Middle East, which has caused a change in the kind of dwelling used in these countries (from open-air, tent-dwellings to air-conditioned skyscrapers which have cool and comfortable rooms, but which are not mold-free).

    b. The forceful displacement through war of millions of people who have been made to move from a dry desert area to a damp area near a seashore where wind currents, climate, and vegetation are ideal for the growth of molds (Israel, Greece, India, etc.).

The Diagnosis of Mold Allergy

Diagnosis of mold allergy rests on an allergic history followed by intracutaneous testing.

Scratch tests are not to be used for molds because they are not reliable. (See Chapter III, *Skin Testing*.) The reading of the test is usually done fifteen minutes after performing it; however, molds are known to cause delayed reactions which show up one or two days after the test. The number of tests necessary to diagnose a mold allergy varies with the training and experience of the allergist who is performing them.

The Treatment of Mold Allergy

Treatment consists of weekly injections of a weak solution of mixed mold extract, to be increased in potency until a maximum tolerated dosage is reached after four to five months. Once that dosage is reached, the period between injections is prolonged until only one injection per month is given for a period of two to three years. These injections provide relief from allergy symptoms in about 80 percent of the mold-sensitive children thus treated. Even in institutes which specialize in mold allergy, the results are not superior.

The list below contains commercial products useful in preventing mold growth in a basement or in other damp areas.

Bye-Mold: Sold by Allergy-Free Products for the Home, Springfield, Missouri.
Impregon: Made by Fleming Company, St. Louis.
Ammonium compounds: Zephiran Chloride, Roccal, and other chlorine solutions, found in drugstores all over the country.
Paraformaldehyde crystals: Two ounces left in an

open jar for several days in a room that is well ventilated prior to reuse.

Formalin (37 percent formaldehyde) : The liquid is to be poured into a wide-mouth container until about one-half inch deep. The number of containers used varies with the size of the basement, and it is most important that the basement be thoroughly aired out before use.

Lysol solution: To use in cleaning the walls and floor of the room.

Electrostatic air purifiers.

Dehumidifiers and desiccants: For example a cloth sack containing two to three pounds of calcium chloride suspended above a pail to collect the drippings.

Incidentals

Incidentals are inhalant allergens that may be incidentally found in a bedroom, even though they may appertain to it naturally. They are a frequent cause of allergy in childhood, ranking next to pollen in their importance.

House Dust

This is a special kind of dust isolated from the inside of a house and recognized as early as 1922 as a potent and common cause of allergy. It is totally different from the dust found in the streets because it is composed of the emanations, the excretions, and the remains of the dead bodies of the common house mite. It may be obtained from a vacuum cleaner whose dust can be purified and used for testing and desensitization.

Precautions Against House Dust

An atopic child should have a room which he uses for sleeping purposes only; he should dress and undress and keep his clothing and books in another room. The bedroom must be made comfortable, pleasant, and colorful, and it must be kept free from dust by using the following precautions.

Cleaning. The room must be vacuumed daily, and it must be given a thorough cleaning once a week: the floor, the furniture, the tops of the doors, the window frames, the sills, etc., must all be cleaned with a damp cloth or oil mop. After the cleaning, the room must have its windows left open for half an hour, and then all doors and windows must be kept closed until the child is ready to occupy the room. If the child must be present in the house during cleaning time, *he must wear a special mask over his mouth and nose.* The best ones are made of polyethylene, which sticks to the skin, does not admit anything except air, and allows the child to talk freely. The dust clinging to it can be washed off later by dipping the mask in water. (See the Appendix.)

Preparation of the bed. The mattress and springs must be cleaned and enclosed in a plastic casing (which may be bought in stores that specialize in allergy-free products). If a second bed must be used in the same room, it must be prepared in the same fashion.

Choice of the bedding material. The pillow must be made of sponge rubber, and the blankets of synthetic material (which is to be

washed every four to six weeks). The bed-
spread must be of washable fabric that has
been laundered previously. *No mattress pad,
quilts, comforters, or fuzzy woolen material is
to be used on the bed.*

The furnishings. They should be simple, not
ornately carved, and should consist of a scrub-
bable wooden chair, cotton curtains (instead of
drapes), and roll-up window shades (instead
of Venetian blinds). All toys present in the
room must be made of wood, rubber, or iron
(instead of stuffed toys which may contain
dust, wool, and molds).

The heating. The temperature must be kept
constantly at about 75°F by means of heated
water and *not heated air.* However, if the room
does have hot air heating, several layers of
cheesecloth must be put on the heat outlets.

The following methods may be used to eliminate dust (as well as other inhalant allergens)
from the air.

Filtration utilizes filters made from paper,
glass wool, etc. The effectiveness of such a
device is contingent upon the type of filter
used, the rate of air exchange, and the size of
the particle to be eliminated. If the size of the
particle is a large one (such as that of a pollen
grain which can measure from twenty to thirty
microns), any simple filtering device fitted into
the bedroom window will do. However, since
most inhalant particles are less than five microns in size (particles of dust, fumes, smoke,
mold spores, bacteria, and viruses), special

material called *Hepa* is necessary to perform the filtration (see the Appendix).

Electrostatic precipitation is achieved with plates charged with a high voltage and put in portable units for bedrooms, or in large units attached to the main ducts of the heating system. These plates attract inhalants and dust particles and precipitate them. The large units do their job well if radiant heat is used; however, with forced hot air heating, conventional filters have to be put in the heating ducts as well. The installation of such devices is becoming less costly each year, and the *expense is tax deductible if they are installed with a doctor's prescription.*

Some Helpful Suggestions To Keep a
Bedroom Free of Inhalant Allergens

1. Never introduce perfume, talc, cosmetics, flowers, mothballs, insect sprays, tar paper, or camphor into the bedroom or its closets.

2. Never store anything under the beds.

3. Enclose any woolen clothes which are kept in the bedroom in a plastic zipper bag.

4. Keep the bed away from a central air-heating outlet (if present).

5. Paint or paper the walls of the room with washable materials (to be inspected at intervals for swellings that may denote a mold collection).

6. Never admit pets with feathers or fur to the bedroom.

7. Never allow smoking in the bedroom.

8. Avoid rugs; instead, install a vinyl floor

(to be wet-cleaned daily and damp-mopped once a week with a solution containing a disinfectant to prevent mold growth).

9. Vacuum the room with a tank-type cleaner; attach a second hose to its outlet and place the end of that hose outside a window to prevent the redistributing of dust. Vacuum the cleaner itself before using it.

Orris Root

Orris is a powder obtained from the root of the iris flower; it was used previously in many kinds of cosmetics because it has a pleasant odor, its color is like that of the human flesh to which it clings firmly, and it holds its scent for a long period of time.

Cosmetics which contain no orris root are advertised as nonallergenic; however, no cosmetic can promise to be totally allergy-free. Commercial sources for orris-free cosmetics include: Elizabeth Arden, Botay, Mary Dunhill, Armand's Sympathy, Max Factor's Pancake, Ar-Ex Cosmetics, Almay, Marcille, Mansfields.

The mother of a child who is sensitive to orris should throw away her old powder puff and should not allow a barber to use any kind of cosmetic powder on the child's head or face after a hair-cutting.

Cottonseed

After cotton is harvested, the fibers are separated from the seeds. The fibers may still contain some seeds, which can cause an extremely dangerous form of allergy. The following should be avoided:

Linters: The short cotton fibers clinging to the seeds and used as stuffing in high-grade mattresses, cushions, upholstery fillings, coarse cotton yarns, and to make miniature golf courses.

Hulls: Used in feeding beef and cattle (milk obtained from cows fed these hulls is a highly dangerous source of cottonseed allergy).

Cake: Used in feeding cattle, as fertilizer, or as flour to make doughnuts.

Oil: Used in making oleomargarine and mayonnaise (in general, this oil is a very weak allergen).

Tobacco

Smoking may create or aggravate existing respiratory allergy because cigarettes may contain (besides tobacco) many potentially allergenic ingredients, such as licorice and molasses.

An allergic person, child or adult, should avoid small rooms and enclosed spaces where crowds gather and smoke (such as the smoking section of movie houses) because hot tobacco smoke is a nonspecific irritant besides being a potential allergen.

Pyrethrum

Pyrethrum is a powder prepared from the dried flower of the pyrethrum plant, which is related to the ragweed plant. It is used as an insecticide to spray plants in backyards or in moth killers to preserve winter clothing and carpeting.

For insecticides free from pyrethrum see the Appendix.

Kapok

These fibers are used for filling life preservers (because they remain afloat for hours without much absorption of water) ; for insulation purposes; and for less expensive sleeping bags and mattresses. (Kapok was used in the past as a filling for pillows to avoid highly allergenic feathers. However, this practice has now stopped because of the development of foam rubber, plastics, and synthetic fibers.) Kapok seeds provide an oil used in making soap and in the preparation of certain foods.

Flax

Flax is the Latin word for the linen plant which provides linseed oil and linen fibers. Linseed oil may cause allergies when eaten, inhaled, or touched, and linen fibers may cause eczema and rashes when they are used in clothing.

Flax fibers, seeds, or oil may be inhaled when one is near flaxseed meal (which is a food given to cattle and poultry) ; in beauty salons and barber shops (as some wave sets, shampoos, and hair tonics (Kreml) may contain it) ; using bird lime, carron oil, flaxseed poultices, furniture polish, linseed oil, paints, varnishes, linoleum, printer's and lithographic ink, some soft soaps, and some depilatories; or

using damask, table linen, cambric, handker-
chief linen, toweling, oilcloth, and sewing
thread.

Epidermoids

The scales, hair, or feathers normally shed by
dogs, cats, horses, goats, rabbits, birds, sheep,
rats, and mice are highly allergenic. Atopic
children are easily sensitized to these skin out-
growths, and they should avoid them regardless
of the results of skin tests.

Dogs sensitize through their hair, saliva, or
dander (scales). Because dander is more allergenic than hair or saliva, allergy to the live animal is more severe than that caused by the
hair of a dead animal used in furs or rugs or
the saliva dripped on floors and furniture.

Allergy to dogs is common because the dog is
a popular domestic pet; however, allergy to one
breed of dog does not necessarily indicate an
allergy to all other breeds. Yet all breeds are
potentially dangerous, and a change in dog
breed is not a solution to dog allergy.

If an atopic child does not have a dog, he
should not get one. If he has one and he is emotionally attached to it, he should be allowed to
keep it, but should not be allowed to replace it
when it dies. Meanwhile, the dog should not en-
ter his bedroom, and it should be kept outside
the house as much as possible.

Even though avoiding dogs may be heart-
breaking for a dog-loving child, there is no solution to this problem at the present time
(except through a prolonged desensitization

program which may not produce satisfactory results). For now, an atopic child should try to live without a dog.

Cats cause allergy because they lend themselves to cuddling and close contact. Their hair is light in weight, and it clings to the furniture for two to three weeks after the cat has been removed from a room. Persons allergic to cats should likewise avoid the other members of the cat family, such as the panther, the lynx, and the leopard (in visits to the zoo).

Commercially, cat hair is used in cheap furs, Chinese rugs, gloves, and toy animals.

Horse hair can be contacted directly through riding or indirectly through contact with the hair clinging to the clothes of persons connected with riding in academies, stables, or racetracks. The stuffing of upholstered furniture and orthopedic mattresses, rope, gloves, toys, fur coats, and suits may contain horse hair and should be avoided. A visit to a zoo should be avoided because the pony, the mule, and the zebra all belong to the horse family.

A person who is allergic to horse hair is usually allergic to horse serum as well. (Horse serum is still used in backward countries to carry tetanus antitoxins.)

Goat hair is known as mohair when it comes from the Turkish goat, alpaca when it comes from the llama of peru, and cashmere when it comes from the goats in India. It is used to make clothing, costly Oriental rugs, imitation astrakhan, Utrecht velvet, cheap blankets, mops, ropes, brushes, and cheap plaster mixes.

Rabbit may cause allergies in children who keep rabbits as pets. Rabbit hair is used to make coats, trimmings, carriage robes, lining for gloves, slippers, food muffs, mattresses, pillow stuffings, quilts, toy animals, infant wear, hand-knitted trimmings, crochet work, gloves, hosiery, and knee pads for invalids and rheumatic children. Rabbit hair made into felt is used in the manufacture of hats, sounding hammers for pianos, insulation material for buildings, polishing pads, washers for cartridges, and insulation material for shoes. Rabbit hair furs used to be sold with deceptive names suggestive of expensive furs. This practice has now been stopped by law.

Birds and their feathers are an important cause of allergy which should be avoided regardless of the results of skin tests. A child should avoid feathers in his bedroom pillow. (The nearness of the nose to the pillow during the prolonged hours of sleep may account for bad allergic symptoms in the nose and lungs. Old feathers are more dangerous than new ones because they gather dust and molds). Allergic children should not keep birds as pets (canaries, parakeets, etc.).

Sheep wool is an outgrowth of the skin of the animal. Because it is warm, flexible, and light, it is the ideal body cover in cold climates and has been used for this purpose for thousands of years.

Allergy to wool is caused mainly by fuzzy woolen blankets and coarse socks. Soft woolen clothing loses much of its allergenic powers through the processing and dyeing of the wool thread. Cloth spun from wool includes albatross, astrakhan, blankets, broadcloth, felt, flannel, gabardine, jersey, rugs, serge, suede, tapestry, mohair, tweed, velour, and whipcord.

Silk is a thread spun by the silkworm and is frequently used to make clothing. Rayon (or artificial silk) is a synthetic product made of cotton; it may be used safely by children who are sensitive to silk.

BACTERIA AND VIRUSES AS ALLERGENS

A newborn baby has antibodies in his blood that protect him against respiratory infections. These antibodies, which he gets from his mother while he is still in the womb, are used up during the first year of life and leave him exposed to infections during the early part of his second year, until he makes enough antibodies of his own. During this interim period, the baby's respiratory infections become frequent and cause inflammations that erode his respiratory mucosa. These erosions permit the passage of minute particles of dead bacteria into his blood. These particles become allergens which cause wheezing in the chest each time the baby is exposed to the same bacteria. Furthermore, an inflamed respiratory mucosa promotes the absorption of inhalant allergens, and the relationship between inhalant allergy and infection becomes very intimate. As a result, infectional allergy acquires these characteristics: it is frequently accompanied by inhalant allergies; a vaccine prepared from the bacteria and viruses of children with infectional allergy and given to them for desensitization purposes at times increases their symptoms; the symptoms of infectional allergy disappear with the use of antibiotics, as well as with the removal of the source of infections in the tonsils and adenoids.

The treatment of infectional allergy rests on four objectives:

a. Arrest of the infection with antibiotics
b. Control of the allergy with conventional remedies
c. Avoidance of the recurrence of the infection by removal of the source of the infection in the tonsils and adenoids
d. Desensitization against bacteria and viruses with cultures taken from the deep tissues of one's own tonsils and adenoids, or with stock vaccines.

Tonsillectomy in an Atopic Child

Tonsils confer immunity to infections and prevent allergy. However, frequent infections in the tonsils clinically cause more allergy when irritants, pollutants, chilling, sweating, or emotional upsets coexist with the infections.

The question arises as to whether one can prevent allergy through the removal of the tonsils (and their bacteria), or whether one should avoid the procedure because it may lower the child's resistance to infection, thus causing more allergies in the long run. The answer lies in the case in question. All the indications for a tonsillectomy are the same whether the child is atopic or not. They are the presence of frequent, repeated, and severe tonsillar infections; an inability to swallow caused by abnormally large tonsils; the presence of a peritonsillar abscess; recurrent, intermittent, or permanent hearing loss. However, should tonsillectomy become imperative in an atopic child, it should be done in a pollen- and mold-free season and in an allergy-free atmosphere. (The operating room, as well as the bedroom of the child, must be equipped with electrostatic air-cleaning devices to avoid exposing the abraded tonsillar area to new inhalants and infectional agents.)

DRUGS AS ALLERGENS

Drugs may be absorbed by mouth, by injection, by inhalation, or by contact. They may be well accepted, or they may cause intolerance or allergy. Intolerance is an exaggerated response to a large quantity of a drug, while allergy is a sensitivity to the drug regardless of the quantity used.

Allergy to a drug assumes one of these forms:

a. A local inflammation and itching (for example, at the site of a penicillin injection)
b. A fixed reaction caused by swelling and

      itching which appears in the same place
each time the drug is used
c. Hives
d. Anaphylaxis
e. Serum sickness

Drug allergy is usually less severe in children than in adults; drugs sensitize when first used, but open the door to dangerous reactions later on. A good example of this is anaphylaxis caused by a second injection of penicillin.

Anaphylaxis
This is a dangerous allergic reaction which may occur after an allergy injection, a bee sting, the eating of allergenic foods, an injection of horse serum, or an injection of penicillin. The symptoms may be shock, hives, congestion in the nose, or asthma. To prevent anaphylaxis, a careful history (to avoid a potential allergen) should be taken by the child's allergist.

A child who has had a slight reaction to penicillin should avoid its use. In case it is imperative to use it, it is much safer to have it taken by mouth than by injection. Furthermore, injections of penicillin are to be given in the arm and not in the buttocks, so that a tourniquet may be placed above the place of the injection to slow down the passing of the injected material into the circulation (in case of a reaction).

The *treatment* of anaphylaxis consists of:

a. An injection of adrenalin to relax the spasm of the bronchi and to diminish the secretions of the mucus glands
b. An intravenous injection of calcium gluconate
c. Monitoring of the blood pressure so that another injection of adrenalin can be given if it becomes necessary
d. Hospitalization

Serum Sickness

An allergic reaction to an injection of horse serum can produce serum sickness. It occurs in 10 percent of children if only 10 cc. of serum are injected, while the incidence rises to 90 percent if 100 cc. are injected. The symptoms are hives, swelling of the joints, and fever. These may appear immediately after an injection, be delayed, or be accelerated. An immediate reaction appears minutes after an injection; a delayed one appears hours after an injection; an accelerated one appears days after the injection.

If a child has had any one of these reactions, a skin test for the serum that has caused the reaction is unnecessary and dangerous. However, if a previous injection went by without a reaction, a skin test for the serum is necessary before giving it again.

In case a child must take a tetanus shot and he is known to be allergic to horse serum, then a human serum which is rich in the same kind of antibodies has to be given to him instead. This serum is to be injected intramuscularly as one single dose. Although human serum has never caused an allergic reaction, this remains a possibility. To avoid it, active immunization against tetanus with toxoids is mandatory to eliminate the need for any tetanus immune serum.

Special precautions are necessary to immunize an egg-sensitive atopic child against influenza, measles, rubella, and mumps vaccines because these vaccines contain egg. (However, if the child has hives or asthma after eating eggs, then *no* egg vaccine is to be given to him).

Flu vaccination must be given in three doses—the second one two weeks after the first, and the third two months after the second, starting in September and going into December. The vaccine used has to be free from alum, be polyvalent, contain the Asian flu virus, and be given intracutaneously in one-tenth of the regular dose.

While giving the atopic child any kind of immunization, a pediatrician should have adrenalin on hand for unforeseen reactions.

Aspirin and Penicillin

Aspirin may cause hives, perennial rhinitis, nose polyps, or asthma. Many salicylates (even though similar in structure to aspirin) may not cause allergic symptoms in an aspirin-sensitive person.

Penicillin allergy is a very serious illness which reflects the amount given, the route of administration, a previous exposure to it, and the presence of an infection. Its incidence among the population of any country may be judged approximately because only its spectacular reactions are noticed, while its minor symptoms may be overlooked and confused with the disease being treated.

One type of allergic reaction to penicillin is the immediate one which may occur a few minutes after ingestion or injection. Its symptoms range from a mild fever to itching, to rashes, to hives, to serum sickness, to asthma, to hemorrhage, to contact dermatitis, or to anaphylactic shock. The second type of reaction is the delayed one which may appear two to three days after contact; it manifests itself as hives, laryngeal edema, or a choking sensation. Lastly, there is an accelerated reaction to penicillin which may occur one week after its contact; this manifests itself as a rash, hemolytic anemia, or pains in the joints.

Children who have never taken penicillin as such may still show an allergy to it if they have drunk milk from cows treated with penicillin; if they have eaten a moldy food; or if they were given immunizations in syringes that have been used to inject penicillin. (Boiling and sterilization do not destroy penicillin or prevent allergy to it.)

3

Skin Testing

If a child is suspected of having allergies, a confirmation is possible through the following means: an allergic history, a physical examination, laboratory tests, a study of the environment, and a diet evaluation. When this workup points toward an allergy, skin tests and a Rast reaction test will detect the cause or causes of the disease.

The Allergic History
An allergic history should be taken by the child's doctor and should include:

Name
Address
Chief complaint
Family history of allergies
Infectious and contagious diseases
Immunizing procedures and reactions
Pets in the house
Bedding (covers, blankets, mattresses, sheets, etc.)
Nose and throat infections (colds, tonsillitis)
Food idiosyncrasies
Present illness:
   Initial attack
   Subsequent attacks
   Last attack
Tentative diagnosis

SKIN TESTING

Once the allergic history and other standard workup procedures are completed, skin testing is begun. This involves the provocation of an allergic reaction in the skin through exposure to a minute amount of an allergen. It is the easiest and simplest method of detecting a sensitivity to an inhalant allergen, but it has little value unless the above-mentioned studies point to it.

One method of skin testing is to first prick or scratch the surface of the skin and then put an allergenic extract on the abraded area. Another method (intradermal) is to introduce, with a needle, a small quantity of an allergenic extract between the layers of the skin. A third method (used to detect the cause of contact eczema) is the patch test, which places a piece of gauze soaked in the suspected allergen on the skin for a prolonged period of time. A fourth method, rarely used now, is the conjunctival test, performed by putting a drop of an allergenic extract in the eye.

All these tests may be performed before, while, or after allergy symptoms are present. However, some drugs used to control allergies, such as antihistamines, adrenalin, aminophylline, atropine, and ephedrine, may reduce the intensity of the skin's reaction to the test. These drugs should be discontinued forty-eight hours before any skin test is performed. (Cortisone, on the other hand, even though very effective for allergies, has no effect on a skin test.)

The skin of the inside of the arm is used for scratch or intradermal tests because the arm allows the use of a tourniquet in case of a severe reaction to testing. To perform scratch tests, a small scalpel which can make an incision in the skin (without drawing blood from it) is used. The skin site is cleaned with alcohol, ten scarifications are made, and a small amount of an allergen extract is placed over each scarification. To perform intradermal tests, the skin site is cleaned with alcohol, a different allergenic extract is put into each one of ten disposable allergy syringes, and an injection of 0.02 cc. of each extract is made between the layers of the skin.

After performing skin tests, an "immediate" reaction may appear after fifteen minutes, or a "delayed" reaction may appear ten to fifteen hours later. (Delayed reactions are known to occur when testing for molds.) These tests are read differently by different allergists. Some doctors consider that:

a. A slight skin reaction is a one-plus reaction.
b. A moderate reaction is a two-plus reaction.
c. A marked reaction in a three-plus reaction.
d. A marked active reaction (or one with "branching" feet) is a four-plus reaction.

Others use a mathematical way of reading the tests, depending on the size of the wheal:

a. ½ cm. is considered a one-plus reaction.
b. 1 cm. is considered a two-plus reaction.
c. 1½ cm. is considered a three-plus reaction.
d. 2 cm. is considered a four-plus reaction.

Still others prefer to measure the intensity of a reaction according to the size of a standard circle:

a. A wheal as large as the head of a pin is a one-plus reaction.
b. A wheal as large as a dime is a two-plus reaction.
c. A wheal as large as a nickel is a three-plus reaction.
d. A wheal as large as a quarter is a four-plus reaction.

Skin testing is a very reliable method of determining the kind, as well as the degree, of sensitivity to an inhaled allergen. Intradermal or scratch tests should be performed in three sessions, one session each week, as it is not advisable to perform more than ten of them each time. A possible schedule of testing might look like the one indicated here.

FIRST SESSION	SECOND SESSION	THIRD SESSION
Trees	Silk	Alternaria
Grasses	Feathers	Aspergillus
Plantain	Dog Hair	Penicillium
Ragweed	Goat Hair	Hormodendron
Dust	Horse Hair	Kapok
Tobacco	Horse Serum	Cottonseed
Pyrethrum	Cat Hair	Flaxseed
Orris Root	Rabbit Hair	

The above tests are to be repeated in different dilutions because the intensity of the reaction to each dilution determines the treatment. A very sensitive child classified as AA can tolerate a much smaller quantity of desensitizing material than someone who has been classified as A, B, C, or D. However, even though testing in different dilutions is a good guide to the strength of the solution to be used in desensitization, it does not indicate the actual amount of discomfort that the allergic child may be suffering.

During skin testing, some highly sensitive children may get hives or shock. If this happens, the doctor should place a tourniquet on the arm above the site of the test (in order to delay the absorption of the testing material) and inject adrenalin in the testing area. This injection may have to be repeated in half an hour.

Skin testing for foods has limited value in

the diagnosis of a food allergy. Consequently, many allergists skip these tests altogether. They rely instead on an accurate history and elimination diets. Those who do tests for foods find that intradermal tests are more accurate than scratch tests, but the possibility of severe anaphylactic reactions while testing for shellfish, nuts, and strawberries are possible.

Skin Tests for Contact Dermatitis

A patch test is performed if a careful history (based on the site of the lesion) offers a clue to the offending agent. The gauze used in testing (which is soaked in the suspected material) is left on the skin for forty-eight to seventy-two hours.

The causes of contact dermatitis include the following materials:

Soaps and detergents: May irritate the hands, fingers, or wrists.

Plants: May touch the hands, forearms, ankles, etc. and create an itch usually followed by a secondary bacterial infection. (Examples include poison ivy, poison sumac, English ivy, and philodendron, as well as such plant derivatives as Japanese lacquer and cashew nutshell oil.)

Textiles: May cause contact allergy where the pressure of the clothing is greatest, such as under a hat band.

Jewelry: May cause contact dermatitis on earlobes, neck, and wrists.

Cosmetics: May cause contact dermatitis on

eyelids, ears, fingers, etc. If the dermatitis is present in the scalp, the cause may be scalp lotions, hair tonics, hair dyes, or shampoos; if it is on the eyelids, the cause may be mascaras and eyebrow pencils; if it is in the armpits, the cause may be deodorants.

The Interpretation of Skin Tests

A positive skin test may mean that the allergy is caused by the allergen used in testing; by an allergen that may cause allergy at a future date; by an allergen which has caused allergy in the past; or by an allergen which is similar to the one causing the positive test. Or it may mean that the positive skin finding is a casual one which is not related to the allergy in question. Therefore, extreme care must be exercised in diagnosing an allergy on the basis of skin test interpretations.

If the allergic history and skin tests are not conclusive, the *Rast test* may be used. This test works on the principle of an allergen reacting with its specific antibody in the blood serum of an allergic patient. It is safe, convenient, accurate, time-saving, and less traumatic than skin testing, but it is costly and not always available.

After the allergic history and the skin or Rast tests have been done, all the positive findings should be recorded in the following summary which must be kept in the physician's records and should also be kept by the school nurse, the camp doctor, and the child's parents.

DIAGNOSTIC SUMMARY

Name	Age
Address	Referred by
Date first seen	Date of report

Chief complaint

Present illness

Past history

Family history

Known clinical disagreements

Known drug disagreements

Physical examination

X-rays of chest

X-rays of sinuses

Positive test:

   Pollen

   Epidermoids

   Foods

   Incidentals

   Molds

   Insects

   Others

   Diagnosis

4

Allergic Diseases

IN THE SKIN, NOSE, AND LUNGS

Allergy may manifest itself in the ways listed below:

a. In the skin as eczema, contact dermatitis, or hives
b. In the nose as seasonal rhinitis (hayfever) or nonseasonal (perennial) rhinitis
c. In the eye as allergic conjunctivitis
d. In the ear as serous otitis media
e. In the sinuses as allergic sinusitis or nose drip

    f. In the lungs as allergic cough or bronchial asthma

    g. In the gastrointestinal tract as canker sores, allergic vomiting, or diarrhea

THE SKIN

Eczema

A skin disorder which starts at two to three months of age is called eczema. It involves inflammation and itching of the cheeks, the neck, the folds of the arms and legs, the wrists, the hands, and the back. It usually lasts about two years and then subsides by itself. Prolonged itching during this period usually causes secondary infections which make the baby fretful and irritable. Sometimes eczema may persist into adult life and cause the skin to become discolored and thick. In an adult, eczema is more difficult to "manage."

Many doctors do not consider eczema an allergic disorder, but rather a disease of an abnormal skin (although children with eczema are likely to develop hayfever and asthma later on in life).

A complication of eczema called *eczema vaccinatum* may occur if a baby who suffers from active eczema is vaccinated against smallpox. To avoid this complication, the baby should not be vaccinated early, and the new method of vaccination developed by Kempe should be used. (The material for this kind of vaccination can be obtained from the Department of

Public Health or from allergy clinics or hospitals.)

Hypoallergenic Feeding

The prevention of eczema is achieved partly through hypoallergenic feedings. For example, an atopic baby should be breast fed. If that is impossible, the baby (until eight months of age) has to be fed a hypoallergenic diet that contains no egg, meat, fish, milk, or orange. The one suggested by the author allows everything outlined here.

Juice: Pineapple juice, grape juice, apricot juice, apple juice, Soya milk (15½ oz.) combined with boiled water (15½ oz.)

Fruits: Pineapple, apple, apricot, plum, prune, banana

Cereals: Cornmeal, rice, hominy, Post Toasties, puffed rice, barley cereal

Meats: Lamb, beef, mutton, lamb chops

Vegetables: Fresh or canned asparagus, lettuce, string beans, white potatoes

Breads: Ry-Krisp

Butter: Substitute salted Crisco

Fat: Pure olive oil.

Flour: Substitute cornstarch, rice, rye, barley flours

Miscellaneous: Karo syrup, unflavored gelatin, hard candy flavored with peppermint or wintergreen— *no soft candy.*

Important: Supplementary synthetic vitamins should be added.

Environmental Control

In order to further provide for the prevention of eczema, the child's environment must be controlled.

a. The bedroom of the baby should be free of dust, feathers, fur, animal hair, fuzzy clothing, and silk.
b. The baby must wear cotton fabrics that have been washed with mild detergents (such as Calgon) and that have been rinsed out thoroughly. Woolen clothing (if unavoidable) should be lined with white cotton cloth.
c. The use of regular soap is to be avoided; an alkali-free soap (see the Appendix) should be used on the baby's skin. His skin must never be scrubbed, but patted dry with clean towels, and open lesions on the skin should not be picked or scratched.
d. The baby must avoid excessive exposure to the sun by the use of sun-screening agents (see the Appendix).

The Treatment of Eczema

Treatment may be specific, through the elimination of suspected foods and desensitization against inhalant allergens, or symptomatic, through local application of wet dressings, lotions, ointments, or medicated tapes on the skin to relieve itching, protect areas from friction, reduce inflammation, and stimulate healing.

The following principles are used in the local "management" of eczema:

a. The more serious the inflammation, the blander the application.
b. The vehicle of an application is as important as the medicine it carries.

c. The appearance of eczema (and not its cause) determines its "management."

Acutely inflamed eczema is to be medicated with wet dressings of normal saline or Burrow's solution (1:20), which provide moisture, a disinfectant, and an astringent effect. Dressings may be applied open to allow water to evaporate and cause cooling and soothing or closed with a cellophane cover to stop evaporation and maintain heat and moisture on the eczema for some time. A wet dressing can be made by placing a solution in a porcelain, enamel, or plastic container, but *not in a copper or aluminum one,* then soaking a cloth (such as a clean old shirt or bed sheeting) in the solution, wringing out the cloth tightly, folding it in six or eight layers, placing it on the affected area, and securing it with a safety pin. As the compress dries out, it is to be removed, rewet, and reapplied, about six times daily for ten minutes each time, using a fresh solution for each application. After the application, the area should be patted dry. If the eczema is on the hands or feet, these should be soaked directly in a pan containing the solution.

Infected eczema must be treated with antibiotics as well as wet dressings. The medicines that may be added to skin applications to achieve protective, softening, anti-infective, or anti-itch effects are antibiotics, hydrocortisone, coal tar, boric acid, zinc oxide, and salicylic acid. Shake lotions, liniments, ointments, and creams are all skin applications which may contain the above ingredients.

Shake lotions are powders suspended in water to be used on scaly patches of skin. Upon evaporation of the water, a thin layer of powder remains on the skin. Liniments are lotions containing an oil; they form the transition between shake lotions and ointments. Ointments are fats containing a medication to soften thick and horny skin and a medication to heal its inner layers. Creams contain water along with fat and medication.

All ointments and lotions are to be used sparingly, as a little dab is just as effective as a larger amount. Each medicated area must be bathed with warm water and an alkali-free soap before every new application.

Medicated cortisone tape, such as Cordran, presents the following advantages over lotions, creams, or ointments. Its application is easy; its penetration is enhanced by an occlusive action which hydrates and softens the skin; it is not bulky (fitting easily under shoes or socks); it is not messy; it protects against scratching; it permits a clean, uniform, and permanent application of medication to a localized area of eczema. There is also no irritation or pain when the tape is peeled off and replaced every twelve hours.

The skin is prepared before the application of the tape by cleaning off scales, crusts, dried exudates, or any previously used ointments or creams with a saline solution. No soap is to be used, and there is no need to remove hair. If an irritation or an infection should occur, the use of the tape should be discontinued.

Large areas of eczema should be treated with baths. Colloidal baths are used for acute eczema. They may consist of:

Bran: Very hot water is allowed to run into a tub over a cheesecloth bag containing one to three pounds of wheat bran. The tub is filled with water, and the bag is squeezed occasionally to introduce the bran into the water.

Cornstarch: One pound of cornstarch is stirred into a tub full of water.

Oatmeal: Two cups of boiled oatmeal are put into a cheesecloth bag, and then the bag is used as a washcloth on the skin. (For ready-made oatmeal mixtures, see the Appendix.)

Tar baths which are helpful in subacute eczema are made with three ounces of a solution of crude coal tar, N.F., put into a full tub of water. (For ready-made tar baths see the Appendix.) Sodium bicarbonate baths are soothing for very irritated and itchy skin. One cup of sodium bicarbonate to a tub of water is used. Magnesium sulfate baths may be used, one cup to a tub of water, for actuely inflamed skin which is oozing.

Failure in the treatment of eczema may be caused by a bacterial or a fungal infection, a concomitant contact dermatitis, seborrhea, an endocrine disturbance, an immunological disorder, a situation of stress, or a drug eruption that takes place at the same time as the eczema.

Tranquilizers are a radical part of the treatment of any form of eczema. Atarax or Vistaril are generally chosen in syrup form to be given by mouth in teaspoonfuls three or four times daily for a period of three to four months.

Contact Dermatitis

This is an inflammation in the skin caused by touching an abrasive chemical or because of allergic sensitivity. (See Chapter II.)

Poison Ivy, Poison Sumac, and Poison Oak Dermatitis

The poison ivy plant is a vine which climbs on trees, hedges, or stone walls and has a leaf composed of three leaflets, two of which are opposite each other. The leaf is about three inches long, and its edges are either smooth or have notches. The plant is green in summer and turns red in the fall. In May and June it bears small clusters of greenish-white flowers which turn into white berries (not poisonous to eat) the size of a raisin during the fall. Its flowers and fruit clusters may remain on its branches after the leaves have fallen.

The poison sumac plant is a coarse woody shrub (which is known as swamp sumac) that never assumes the vine-like form of poison ivy. Its leaves are divided into from seven to thirteen pairs of leaflets, with a single leaflet at the end of the stem.

Poison oak (otherwise known as oak-leaf ivy) is a low-growing shrub which has slender, upright branches that bear leaflets similar to those of the oak tree and fruits similar to those of the poison ivy plant.

An unseen oil which coats the leaves of all of these plants may stick to the hands, shoes, or clothes of the person who touches them and may remain there for many months (strongly enough to revive the dermatitis). Smoke from a burning poison ivy plant may carry enough of this oil to cause irritation in the nose or eyes of a person standing in the vicinity of the fire.

The symptoms of poison ivy dermatitis are a slight redness in the skin followed by a mild itch which slowly increases in intensity. The redness may turn into tiny watery blisters after a few hours. These may burst, ooze, dribble over the skin, and become infected. The oozing material, however, does not spread the disease to other parts of the body or to other people. The blisters take about two weeks to heal without any medication.

Treatment of poison ivy dermatitis consists of washing the affected skin *immediately* with soap and water (to stop the oil from reaching the deep layers of the skin). If blisters have already formed, dressings of normal saline should be applied. If the blisters have become infected, the application should be tepid soaks of 1:10 Burrow's solution. Antihistamines may also be used if local applications fail to bring relief. In severe cases, the only treatment that may help is prednisone taken by mouth.

A child should be taught the following:

    a. To identify poison ivy, poison sumac, and poison oak leaves

    b. That he should immediately wash the area that has touched the plants with soap and water

    c. That poison ivy dermatitis may occur at any time during the year by contact with twigs of the dormant plant, but that the danger is greatest in spring and summer when the oil of the plant is abundant and lively

    d. That poison ivy dermatitis is not necessarily an allergic disease and that any child may get it

    e. That he may get poison ivy dermatitis by touching clothes or animals that have been contaminated with it, by inhaling the smoke of the burning plant, or by eating the buds of the plant

Hives or Urticaria

Hives is an illness characterized by itchy wheals on the skin accompanied, at times, by fever and nausea. It may be acute and last a few hours to a few days or chronic and last months or years. Its common causes are foods (fish, chocolate, nuts, cantaloupe, and corn), drugs (penicillin and aspirin), bee and insect bites, worms in the stool, bacteria in decayed teeth or infected gallbladders, and emotion. Its prevention is through avoidance of such sensitizing foods, drugs, infections, or emotional stress. Treatment (in acute hives caused by a food) is a light purge, to be followed by an allergy-free diet for a few days. In any other form of acute hives, adrenalin and antihistamines have to be used. Chronic hives respond to the long-range use of tranquilizers (see the Appendix). Steroids in the treatment of hives should be reserved only for refractory cases that have not responded to the above treatments.

Unusal Forms of Hives

Hives may be caused by allergy to a physical agent such as cold, sunlight, or mechanical pressure. This is proven by the fact that many children who suffer from this kind of allergy have a family history of other allergic disorders as well; that generalized hives may occur even after local exposure to a physical agent; that a gradual desensitization against the causative allergens (with repeated exposure to the physical agent) is possible; that antiallergic drugs (such as antihistamines) provide relief in this type of hives.

Cold may cause hives after cold showers, after touching ice cubes, or after bathing in the ocean. Accidental drownings have been related frequently to severe systemic reactions caused by massive histamine release while a person is swimming. Children with this sensitivity have to be desensitized against cold by plunging their hands into water that is 50°F. (Use a thermometer to check the temperature of the water.) The first week this must be done twice daily for one minute; the second week, twice daily for two minutes; the third week, twice daily for three minutes; the fourth week, twice daily for four minutes; the fifth week, twice daily for five minutes. If by the fifth week of treatment there is no improvement, the period of desensitization has to be increased by one minute each day until the child's hands are submerged ten minutes per bath twice a day. If no relief is forthcoming, treatment has to be discontinued.

Sunlight may bring about urticaria caused by ultraviolet rays. The swelling and redness of this urticaria are present in the exposed skin; that is, on every part of the body except under the bathing suit. Sun-screening oils must be used before exposure, and antihistamines are also helpful if taken beforehand (see Appendix).

Overeating, gluttony, and excitement may cause hives by promoting the absorption of foods which are not properly digested.

Horse serum used in the treatment of tetanus may cause hives one week after the injection.

Inhalants (dust, molds, or pollen) may cause hives, a condition which usually responds to desensitization.

Allergies to Bees and Insects

The sting of a bee may cause dangerous allergic reactions in an atopic child. The symptoms vary according to the amount of venom injected, the presence of sensitivity, and the place of the sting.

A normal reaction consists of the formation of a wheal, irritation, itching, and local heat.

The reaction disappears without treatment three or four hours after the sting.

An exaggerated reaction consists of an intense local redness that lasts for one or two days and disappears with cold compresses and an antihistamine.

A toxic reaction is brought about by multiple bee stings which cause poisoning and not allergy. Symptoms are diarrhea, vomiting, fainting, and possibly death (although some children are known to have survived as many as a thousand bee stings).

A serum-sickness-like reaction consisting of generalized hives and inflammation in some joints may appear one or two weeks after a sting.

Anaphylactic shock, which occurs two or three minutes after the sting, may consist of a dry cough, a sense of constriction in the throat, a massive eruption of hives, a drop in blood pressure, and a constellation of other symptoms (vomiting, chills, involuntary bowel movements, confusion, collapse, and death).

Hyposensitization

The prevention of bee stings can be achieved by teaching the child to:

a. Avoid food that is discarded in outside garbage cans.
b. Avoid gardens (because flowers attract bees and vines conceal their nests).
c. Avoid clothes with bright, flowery prints, for they, too, attract bees.

d. Wear shoes when outdoors.
e. Take vitamin B1 during the summer (it gives an odor to the body which bees avoid).

Children who are known to be allergic to bees should be desensitized with a mixture of bee, wasp, hornet, and yellow jacket antigens

Other insects such as the ant, mosquito, bedbug, flea, spider, tick, mite, and scorpion may cause allergic reactions. They can be avoided with house screens, or discouraged with repellents. The U.S. Department of Agriculture, Bureau of Entomology, Washington, D.C., is ready to give advice on the eradication of any one of these insects.

The eradication of bee hives from an area has to be done by a professional exterminator who should inspect the premises at weekly intervals during the spring and summer to detect budding hives. Wasps build hives in almost any protected place, and their nests can be destroyed by hosing them or knocking them down with a stick or broom handle. Spraying the area with an insecticide discourages them from rebuilding in the same place. Yellow jackets build hives in the ground and emerge through a small hole which should be marked. At dust (after all the insects have returned for the night), gasoline, which need not be lighted, should be poured down the hole. Hornets build nests in the branches of tall shrubs or trees.

Allergic children going to camp should carry an emergency kit containing 10 mg. Isuprel tab-

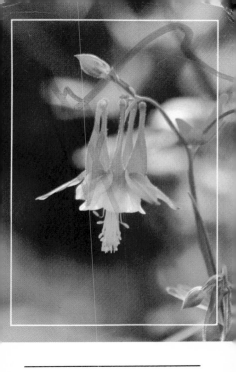

As for man,
his days are
as grass:
as a flower
of the field,
so he flourisheth.

Psalm 103:15

Pictorial by W. J. Bosche Jr.
© 1979 Concordia Publishing House

No. 39-2130
Printed in USA

lets, an adrenalin aerosol (for inhalation), a tourniquet, a pair of tweezers (for the removal of the stinger and venom sac), and an antiseptic towel.

The child should be taught to immediately remove the bee stinger and its sac with the tweezers (particularly in a sting by a honey bee, instant removal of the stinger and sac may help prevent the poison from being absorbed into the blood); to suck one tablet of Isuprel under the tongue; to use the adrenalin inhaler if there is difficulty in breathing; to apply a tourniquet on the arm above the sting site; to clean the sting site with an antiseptic towel; to apply a cold pack to the sting area; to take an antihistamine by mouth; and to contact the nearest doctor or hospital as soon as possible.

THE NOSE AND SINUSES

The nose cleans the air on its way to the lungs by trapping particles that may be suspended in it and by expelling them with mucus in a sneeze. Some particles may remain in the nose and cause a nonseasonal allergy called perennial allergic rhinitis, or a seasonal allergy called hayfever.

Perennial Rhinitis

This comes about when allergenic particles of dust, feathers, animal dander, or wool dissolve in the mucus of the nose and cause stuffiness, sneezing, itching in the palate, throat, and ears, rubbing of the nose, nose wrinkling, mouth breathing, sniffling, a nasal twang, and dark shadows under the eyes. (Many conditions besides allergy may cause a stuffed nose, such as hypothyroidism, abuse of nose drops, viral infections, foreign bodies in the nose, a deviated septum, or abnormal sensitivity to quick changes in temperature, altitude, and stress.)

Treatment of perennial rhinitis is through desensitization, diet, and environmental control, all of which are discussed elsewhere in this book.

The drugs to use in treatment are antihistamines and ephedrine, taken by mouth or in nose drops and sprays. However, *the use of such drops and sprays should be limited to two weeks,* because longer periods of use may irritate the mucosa of the nose and result in bad closure of the nostrils.

To give nose drops to a baby, hold the infant's head as far back as possible with the left hand (keeping the right arm quiet). Put the drops in each nostril every three to four hours. For nursing infants, the drops have to be put in fifteen minutes before feeding time.

For older children, let the head of the child hang downwards off a bed. While he is in this position, turn his head to the right and put the drops in his left nostril. Leave him in this position for ten or fifteen seconds, then turn his head to the left, put the drops in his right nostril, and again leave him in this position for ten to fifteen seconds.

Hayfever

Hayfever is a seasonal inflammation of the nose and eyes caused by allergy to pollen or molds. In the United States, about ten percent of hayfever patients suffer from allergy to tree pollen; thirty percent suffer from allergy to grass pollen; and sixty percent suffer from allergy to weed pollen. The most characteristic feature of hayfever is its periodicity: it recurs each year in the season of pollination of the plant or the sporulation of the mold that causes the allergy. The seasons of plant pollination are different in different areas of the country. A state-by-state listing, giving the months of pollination of trees, grasses, or weeds, is to be found in the Appendix.

Hayfever is a disease that affects a total of five to ten percent of the population of the United States. It begins in early childhood (usually after the age of three), and whether a child gets it or not is determined by heredity and by the amount of pollen or molds he inhales. However, fatigue, exertion, infection, and emotional stress contribute to its early development. Boys and girls develop it equally, but the black and yellow races seem to develop it less than the white race, and the full-blooded American Indian does not seem to develop it at all. The disease is found all over the world, but it is most frequent in the temperate zone.

Hayfever symptoms appear in the early hours of the morning as sneezing, nasal obstruction, a profuse watery discharge from the

nose, a sensation of heat and fullness in the
eyes, a discharge of a copious fluid from the
eyes, a huskiness of the voice, fatigue, loss of
appetite, restlessness, profuse perspiration, a
quickening of the pulse, a dry and irritating
cough, headaches, slight temperature elevation,
and general discomfort and nervousness.

The following conditions are necessary for
any kind of pollen or mold to be accepted as a
cause of hayfever:

    a. The pollen or mold should cause the disor-
       der when brought in contact with the nose.
    b. The disorder should show itself only when
       the specific pollen or mold is abundant in
       the air.

The treatment of hayfever is

Preventive: By avoidance of the specific pollen through the use of a mechanical filtering
device or an electrostatic precipitator in the
bedroom; by sending the child to a pollen-free
area; and by keeping the child indoors as much
as possible during the pollen season.

Symptomatic: With antihistamines.

Specific: Through desensitization which is to
be started three months before the season of
the pollen and given throughout the entire
year, if that is possible.

The prevention of hayfever is made more
complete by:

    a. Removing all flowers, trees, grasses, or
       weeds from the backyard.
    b. Having the child avoid flowers which are
       members of the ragweed family, such as as-

ters, bachelor's buttons, calendulas, chrysan-
themums, cosmos, dahlias, daisies, dande-
lions, marigolds, sunflowers, zinnias, golden-
rod, or any other type of flower in full
bloom.

c. Being aware that dust (originating in long-
time closed trunks, attics, oll books, old pillows, old mattresses, woolens, and cottons),
cosmetics (highly scented toilet articles, nail
lacquer, lacquer removers, hair tonics),
chemical fumes (floor wax, gasoline, insecticides, dry-cleaning fluids, fumigating gases,
moth preventives, and tobacco smoke),
strong light rays (near the sea or in motion
picture houses), and chlorine (in swimming
pools) may cause symptoms similar to those
of hayfever.

Sinusitis

Sinuses are large hollow spaces containing
air found in the bones of the face. They are
covered with a hairy lining that secretes mucus
which drains through natural openings into the
nasal cavities. The sinuses above the eyes are
called frontal sinuses. Those under the eyes are
maxillary sinuses. The ethmoidal sinuses are
above the nose cavities, and the sphenoidal
sinuses are deep inside the skull. Their function is to warm and moisten the air that one
breathes, to lessen the weight of the bones of
the skull, and to contribute to voice resonance.
Sinuses continue to develop until puberty.

When the opening between a sinus and the
nasal cavities becomes blocked, the air in the
sinus is absorbed into the blood. Lack of air
creates a vacuum in the cavity, causing severe

pain that normally develops in mid-morning and eases toward evening. The pain becomes worse when the child bends over, shakes his head, or presses his eyes.

Allergies or a bacterial inflammation may block the natural openings of the sinuses. An upper respiratory infection, a tooth abscess draining into the sinus cavity, a deviated septum, polyps, or enlarged adenoids can all cause bacterial inflammation and blockage.

Sinus blockage is encouraged by polluted city air, vitamin deficiencies, hypothyroidism, chlorine irritation, and travel in pressurized airplanes.

Prevention and Treatment of Sinusitis

The air in a house may be excessively heated in winter. It becomes dry and acts as a sponge, soaking up the moisture of the skin and the lining of the nose, throat, sinuses, and lungs. As a consequence, mucus in the respiratory tract becomes thick and infected.

The amount of moisture in the air as compared to the amount it can hold is called its relative humidity. The ideal relative humidity of a heated house whose indoor temperature is between 60° and 70°F is 50 percent; however, most American homes have a relative humidity in winter of about 14 percent, which is supplemented with vapor from large humidifiers that have an automatic control (cold water vapor provides better results than hot water vapor; see Appendix). Pans of boiling water in different rooms of the house cannot serve the purpose of constant and controlled humidification.

In summer, the situation may be reversed; excessive humidity can be controlled by installing a dehumidifier. There are many excellent units on the market suitable for a private home, an apartment, or both.

The treatment of sinusitis depends on its cause, which may be allergy, infection, or both.

Allergic sinusitis is characterized by sneezing, a watery flow from the nostrils, clogging of the nose, a history of allergy, polyp formation, and a nasal smear that contains eosinophiles. Its treatment is specific through testing and desensitization and nonspecific with decongestants.

Infective sinusitis is characterized by a foul odor in the nose, temperature elevation, pain in the sinus region, a discharge of pus from the sinus opening, and response to antibiotics. Measures to ensure sinus drainage after the passing of the acute infection imply control of the allergy, removal of large adenoids that may hamper sinus drainage, and the avoidance of exposure to further respiratory infections.

Chronic sinusitis may cause anatomical changes in the nose and sinus linings that can make drainage of the sinuses impossible. Surgical procedures (to be done preferably in winter, and, if possible when snow is on the ground) are used to establish new drainage pathways. Puberty may improve chronic sinusitis because obstructing adenoids may become smaller with age.

The Nose Drip of the Allergic Child

Mucus originating in the nose or sinuses is eliminated by filaments (cilia) which are attached to their mucosa. These filaments push the mucus toward the esophagus with a beating movement. However, when the mucus becomes thick and abundant, it is too heavy for the filaments to push back. It remains in place and forms beads that drop on the lungs causing an irritative cough.

The conditions that cause the mucus to be thick and abundant are allergies, low-grade infections, irritants such as tobacco smoke, excessive dryness in the air of the house, overuse of nose drops, emotional disturbances (which affect the sympathetic nervous system and cause an increase in nasal secretions), mechanical obstructions to the drainage of the sinuses (because of a deviated septum or enlarged adenoids), and endocrine deficiencies (such as hypothyroidism, which causes dry, thick mucus formation).

A nose drip is to be "managed" by treating the underlying allergies and by softening the mucus through the use of drops of a saturated solution of potassium iodide (so-called KI) given by mouth. The child should also sleep on high pillows to drain the mucus of the sinus mechanically. A cold air vaporizer should be installed in the bedroom during winter.

The Eye and the Ear in Nose Allergy

The eye becomes involved in allergy of the

respiratory tract because the tear ducts drain into the nose. It follows that an inflammation of the nose spreads easily to the eye.

Vernal conjuctivitis is one form of eye allergy frequently seen in summer among male children in warm climates. Its symptoms are a fear of light, tearing, and a burning sensation in the eye. Its diagnosis is possible because of its seasonal occurrence and because of the cobblestone aspect of the conjunctiva. Treatment consists of corticosteroid drops in the eye (one drop of one percent hydrocortisone solution three to four times daily for one or two weeks). If this is not sufficient, corticosteroids have to be given by mouth.

A tube that connects the middle ear to the pharynx may become clogged by an allergic inflammation. This could cause *a hearing loss* by preventing the drainage of mucus from the middle ear to the pharynx. The treatment consists of ventilation of the middle ear with decongestants and antihistamines; eradication of the infection with antibiotics; suction of the fluid from the middle ear; removal of enlarged tonsils or adenoids; control of the allergies through diet, environmental control, desensitization, and corticosteroids; and respiratory vaccines to prevent recurrent infections.

THE LUNGS

The respiratory tract is made up of large tubes which divide into smaller ones until these become finer than threads. Each tiny tube then ends in a sac where air comes in contact with thin-walled blood vessels to exchange oxygen for the carbon dioxide in the blood. Oxygen cannot be stored in the body; it has to be provided through the air that one breathes, about one-fifth of which consists of oxygen.

Oxygenation and Environment

An altitude of 300 to 600 feet is ideal for healthful oxygenation. (Altitudes above 4,000 feet have less oxygen in the air.)

A warm, dry climate permits outdoor living; it causes fewer lung infections than a rainy, damp climate that requires indoor living. Smoke, dust, fumes, odors, and gases cause fine particles of ash to deposit themselves on the lung mucosa and bring about an extra secretion of mucus which may become infected. Recurrent infections cause a destruction of the air sacs of the lung, a condition called pre-emphysema. This is a ballooning of the chest through air retention. The lungs lose their elasticity and cannot stretch to receive fresh air or recoil to expel stale air.

The diagnosis of pre-emphysema rests on frequent upper respiratory infections, mucus production, a history of breathlessness, wheezing after walking or playing, an X-ray finding in the lung, and a diminished breathing capacity when respiratory function tests are performed.

Preventive measures consist of avoiding upper respiratory infections, removing dust from the bedroom (with an electrostatic precipitator or a filter), and eliminating cigarette smoke from the house.

Drugs which facilitate breathing, such as adrenalin, aminophylline, steroids, antibiotics, expectorants, aerosols of mucolytic agents, saturated solution KI, all help in the treatment of pre-emphysema. Mechanical devices can be used to force oxygen into the lungs, and breathing and postural exercises can help empty the mucus accumulated in the lungs. Two mechanical devices to supplement the lack of oxygen in the lungs are a portable oxygen tank and an intermittent positive pressure machine which can push air forcefully on and off into the alveoli.

Pre-emphysema is a milder illness than emphysema because it is reversible. There are many places in the United States where the outdoor climate is ideal for the healthful breathing of a child with pre-emphysema; for example, Arizona, New Mexico, California, Texas, and Colorado.

The problem of air pollution is recognized universally now, but appropriate solutions come slowly. Air chemistry is in the early stages of scientific development, with government and industry subsidizing dozens of research projects to explore the relationship between environmental, industrial, and automotive emissions and to establish better air quality standards.

Bronchial Asthma

Many diseases of the chest bring about wheezing and difficulty in breathing. Examples of such diseases are allergy, chronic bronchitis, foreign bodies in the lungs, pre-emphysema, enlarged glands, and tumors in the chest.

When wheezing and difficulty in breathing are episodic, bronchial asthma is the cause. Bronchial asthma may be brought about by:

a. Allergy
b. Irritation of the mucosa of the lungs
c. Aspirin
d. Prolonged exercise
e. A combination of factors

To diagnose the cause of bronchial asthma, a doctor needs chest X-rays, a laboratory workup, and a diary which should delineate the weather conditions each day (temperature, humidity, cloudiness, sunshine, smog, rainfall), the symptoms of the illness each day (shortness of breath, wheezing, coughing), the general daily activity, the medications used during the day, any unusual events that have happened each day (exams, a party, etc.), and a list of all the foods eaten by the child that day.

Symptoms can be mild, moderate, or severe. Shortness of breath is mild if the child can carry on his normal routine even though his breathing may be difficult; moderate if the child is able to breathe while lying down but is unable to do any physical work; and severe if he can breathe only while in the sitting position. Wheezing is mild if it can be heard by placing the ear of a stethoscope over the chest; it is moderate if it can be heard from a distance of three feet; and it is severe if it can be heard from another room. The cough is mild if it is easy and productive; moderate if it is difficult and sporadic; severe if it is continuous.

Allergic Asthma

The acute attack of allergic (or extrinsic) asthma is an episodic shortness of breath which lasts hours or days and varies from a tightness in the chest to a severe difficulty in breathing, accompanied by wheezing sounds in the lungs. It may develop suddenly; it may be accompanied by a cough which produces thick mucus; and it may cause breathing which is easy in inspiration but difficult in expiration. Prolonged coughing spells may cause vomiting of food and mucus. Between attacks, the child may be free of symptoms, or he may suffer from spells of coughing and difficulty in breathing.

The attack becomes chronic if the above symptoms continue for a few days in which mild activity and minor events (such as laughing) may be enough to start a new strong attack.

The acute attack becomes *status asthmaticus* if it is not relieved by the conventional asthma drugs. The child becomes apprehensive and agitated; he leans forward in his bed, sweats, and strains to expand his chest; he has a quick heartbeat and a wheezing sound in the lungs that one can hear at a distance; his chest becomes inflated; and his breath sounds are diminished.

Allergic asthma may be caused by foods such as nuts, shellfish, eggs, chocolate, fresh fruit, and mustard; by inhalants such as pollen, house dust, epidermoids, and molds; by drugs; and by bacteria and viruses.

A special kind of asthma caused by molds has certain characteristics which distinguish it from other types of asthma. It has a dramatic onset at night. The child wakes up short of breath, livid, and panicky, but with very little wheezing in his chest. Or it may happen during any day of the year, provided that day has been sunny and warm. The child is free of symptoms when snow is on the ground because snow covers the soil and prevents the mold spores from rising into the air. It is also connected to the eating of mold-containing foods such as Chinese sauces or blue, Roquefort, or Camembert cheeses or to the drinking of any kind of beer fermented with yeast. It is frequent among children of farmers because manure, compost, dead leaves, and musty hay harbor molds.

The advent of air travel (causing extreme changes in the climatic environment), the increase of intermarriage, the use of molds as drugs (penicillin), and the frenzied pace of modern life all contribute to an increase in this kind of asthma.

Nonallergic Asthma

Nonallergic (intrinsic) asthma comes about when a spasm in the muscles of the bronchi occurs after irritants such as cold, damp air, or air containing fumes, tobacco smoke, insecticides, perfumes, and sprays succeed in breaking a child's asthma threshold. An asthma threshold is a theoretical line of defense against spasm situated in the sensory nerve endings lying under the mucosa of the lungs.

Mixed asthma is both allergic and nonallergic at the same time; aspirin asthma is neither allergic nor nonallergic. (See the Appendix for drugs containing aspirin.)

Management of Asthma in Children

There is no "cure" for asthma. We speak of its "management;" that is, the direction of its course until it is relieved or eliminated.

1. Allergic asthma is a simple asthma to manage. Its changes are reversed with adrenalin, with the removal of its cause, and with desensitization.

2. Asthma caused by allergy and infection is more difficult to manage because infections sustain the attacks.

3. Asthma caused by infection alone is even more difficult to manage because there is no allergic factor to remove. The results in its management are usually poor.

4. No improvement can be expected in asthma if the fibrous tissues of the lung have been destroyed.

The following principles must *precede* the prescription of drugs:

An asthmatic child should live in a dry new house because damp old houses have an abnormally high content of house dust and molds.

Ample rest, regular hours for meals, sufficient vitamin intake, and feeding of proper foods are important. Some foods (ice-cold drinks, spicy foods, beans, cabbage, cauliflower, cucumbers, onions, radishes, melons, and turnips) decrease the amount of air that one breathes because they form gases which press on the diaphragm and interfere with its natural movements. Constipation, likewise, causes the full bowels to press against the diaphragm and block its free movement.

Extreme physical fatigue is to be avoided; however, the regular trend of life and its joys must continue. An asthmatic child may ride a bicycle, swim, and participate in competitive games while avoiding his allergens. In bad weather, gymnasiums can be used, provided the child wears a special mask to protect himself from sudden temperature changes when going in and out of the heated gym.

An asthmatic should keep himself busy with hobbies, being careful to adapt them to his condition. If his hobby is building model airplanes and he is allergic to the usual glue, he may substitute vegetable glue. If wool bothers an asthmatic girl and she likes to knit, she can do so by using acrylic instead.

In high school, the asthmatic should participate in all physical activities if that is possible.

Later, after finishing high school, he must choose a college suited for his purposes: he will not be able to perform heavy physical work; inhale dust; be exposed to animals and manure; or smell cosmetics and drugs. Avoiding professions which involve these things will not bring his world to an end; there are many other professions such as general medicine, law, etc., that would enable him to earn a good living.

The asthmatic must be made to remember that he is only one of about nine million children in the United States who have asthma, and that many well-known people had asthma as children. Keeping up his morale is important because anxiety caused by emotional fatigue is exhausting (unpleasant arguments, thriller movies, and fearful television programs are to be avoided as much as possible).

Drugs and Allergic Asthma

Drug management of asthma plays an important role because it provides quick results and permits a desensitization program to work. The drugs used must be simple and have no side effects. Adrenalin, ephedrine, isoproterenol (otherwise called iso), theophylline, and its derivative aminophylline, are all used.

Adrenalin is derived from the suprarenal gland. It is the master drug for acute asthma attacks because it acts quickly, which may be life saving. *The parents of an asthmatic child should know how to give an adrenalin injection:* use a disposable syringe and needle; wipe an area of the outer part of one arm of the child and the top of the adrenalin vial with alcohol; draw the required amount of adrenalin from the bottle and push out the extra air; go through the skin at an angle of forty-five degrees; gently draw back on the plunger, and, if no blood is drawn, inject the adrenalin. If any blood is drawn, withdraw the needle and use a different area for the injection. A 10cc. vial of adrenalin 1:1000 should be kept ready, in the dark, and in a refrigerator. A doctor's prescription is necessary for the adrenalin and the disposable syringe.

Isoproterenol (iso) is a chemical which acts like adrenalin. It comes in a tablet form which is to be put under the tongue (where it dissolves and is quickly absorbed) or as a syrup.

Ephedrine is a plant of Chinese origin that acts like a weak form of adrenalin. It does not stop attacks, but it may help in moderate asthma if used for long periods of time.

Theophylline and its derivative *aminophylline* are very effective bronchodilators which can be given orally, intravenously, or rectally. Intravenously, they should be pushed slowly into the system over a ten-minute period. Rectally, they may be given as an enema or as a suppository containing 250 mg. of theophylline (which is an average child dosage). All theophylline preparations are inherently long acting and should be given at eight-hour intervals instead of the usual three hours allotted for adrenalin.

Other helpful drugs used in asthma include the following:

Steroids: Potent antiallergy drugs derived from two endocrine glands—the pituitary and the adrenal. They can be used for short periods of time only because of their potential hazards: masking infections; increasing fatality rate during surgery; softening the bones; and causing stomach ulcers, high blood pressure, sugar in the urine (not true diabetes), hirsuteness (increase in the growth of hair), increased appetite, an unusual fat distribution in the face (which becomes round and moonlike), depression, and temporary suppression of the natural growth of the bones of a child. All these ill effects disappear when the hormones are discontinued, provided they have been used in small amounts and for a short period of time.

Expectorants: Used to promote coughing and to dislodge the phlegm in the lungs by softening it. Water by mouth, steam by inhalation, and cough mixtures all promote expectoration (which is very important in asthma); cough medicine should never suppress the act of coughing in asthma.

In chronic asthma, drops of the saturated solution of potassium iodide (KI) reduce thick mucus to a soft and watery liquid. It is to be taken by mouth for three to four months, always mixed with milk or juice (in order to mask its taste). The following is one way to prescribe it: The first day the child takes one drop in a teaspoon of milk four times, after meals. Each day after the dosage is increased by one drop daily, until a maximum of ten drops four times a day is reached. On the eleventh day, the reverse process is begun, with nine drops taken four times daily. Each day after the dosage is *decreased* by one drop until one drop is reached again on the nineteenth day. After this, the process starts all over again, first increasing and then decreasing the dosage. The maximum dosage for a child is one drop per year of age from a fresh supply of KI (a ten-year-old child's maximum dosage is ten drops, four times daily).

Possible side effects of potassium iodide are a brassy and burning taste in the mouth and throat, soreness of the teeth and gums, increased salivation, some sneezing, with irritation in the eyes and swelling of the eyelids, headaches, skin rashes, stomach disturbances, drug fever, and, occasionally, goiter. All these side effects cease within a few days after stopping the medication except for goiter, which may last up to two months. If KI drops cause vomiting, the child can take Organidin instead (a child ten years old takes ten drops, four times daily, or one tablet, four times daily).

Antibiotics: Necessary whenever an asthma attack lasts longer than two days. The safest antibiotic is erythromycin; *the most dangerous one is penicillin.*

Aerosols: Jets of gas that carry a medicine reduced into particles. If the particles are large in size, they can be pushed only to the trachea; if they are medium size, they can be pushed to the bronchi; if they are small, they can be pushed to the alveoli. The gas may be compressed air, oxygen, helium, or freon; the propelling apparatus may be a hand nebulizer, an oxygen tank, an air compressor, a special freon cartridge, or an intermittent positive pressure machine. The drugs may be bronchodilators, detergents, enzymes, or antibiotics.

Hospitalization

A mother should not waste her time trying to fight off her child's asthma attack. She should put him to sleep in a dust-free bedroom that contains no animals, feathers, or odors, and give him large quantities of fluids to drink, together with an antihistamine cough mixture that does not contain any codeine. If the attack is strong, she should give him an aminophylline preparation by mouth or rectally. If three hours pass and the attack does not subside, she should give the child an injection of adrenalin which can be repeated in three hours. Any asthma attack that lasts more than a couple of days needs an antibiotic.

Asthma is considered "high risk" and should be treated in a hospital setting *if* the following conditions are present: recurrent *status asthmaticus,* early onset of asthma associated with eczema, dependence on aerosol bronchodilators, congenital chest deformity, living under unfavorable personal surroundings, absence from school for more than one month each year, aspirin intolerance, undiagnosed food or chemical sensitivity, pre-emphysema.

While in the hospital, the asthma attack usually improves dramatically in twenty-four to
forty-eight hours because a change in the
physical environment takes place as well as an
easing of tensions.

Body and Mind in Asthma

Emotions influence bodily health because mind
and body work together as one unit and not
as two separate entities. Emphasis on the
physical aspects in the diagnosis and treatment
of asthma has come about because the emotional factors are difficult to define and are often misleading.

Asthma comes about through a predisposition caused by constitution, heredity, frequent
respiratory infections, and exposure to allergens; once this predisposition has been es-
tablished, an asthma attack may be caused by
allergic factors, by emotional factors, or by a
combination of both. If the emotions are
strong, they may blur the allergic picture and
become the main cause of asthma. As a consequence, asthma caused by allergy and complicated by emotions needs two approaches in its
treatment: a physical one for the changes
brought about by allergy and a psychiatric one
to soothe the emotions (the purpose is to
"cure" the whole child and not just his
asthma).

Psychiatry uses a wide range of procedures
from guidance to reassurance, to analysis, to
group therapy. Regardless of the method used,
an effort would have to be made to understand

the personality structure of the child in order to discover the relationship between his thoughts and acts and how they are influenced by his illness. The purpose of psychiatry would then be to establish maturity, insight, a strengthened ego, and an increase in personal security.

Parentectomy is a long separation of an asthmatic child from his parents. Children who need parentectomy usually come from broken homes in which love and attention to the needs of a sick child are missing; they bring on illness in an unconscious attempt to soothe their emotional needs, while their parents compensate for their guilty feelings by overmedication.

In parentectomy, children are made to live outside their homes for two years with a normal family who will provide them with the love and support they are lacking. During these two years, the parents must obtain family counseling in order to have a more relaxed atmosphere in the house when the child returns.

Hypnosis was a useful tool in the treatment of chronic asthma before the discovery of corticosteroids and tranquilizers because it eased the anxieties that usually accompanied it. Today, it has lost its importance because it is a lengthy and costly procedure that cannot alter an immunological state.

Rehabilitation Homes for Chronic Asthma

Denver has one of the largest institutes in the United States operating under the principle of parentectomy in their asthma rehabilitation

program. There are many excellent asthma institutes throughout the country, in most major cities. Some of them do not require the child to live in, but try to provide help on an out-patient basis. These centers may set up small groups for weekly classes in physical fitness. The age limit is usually from six to sixteen, with groups selected according to age and severity of asthma. (For names of some residential centers see the Appendix.)
Breathing exercises taught in these centers seek to:

    a. Teach the best use of respiratory muscles, especially the diaphragmatic muscle
    b. Teach how to use exercises to stop an asthma attack in its early stages
    c. Improve on exercise capacity
    d. Develop self-confidence

Breathing exercises (see the Appendix) are not curative. They represent only one additional tool to use in the management of asthma.

The Asthmatic Child at Camp and School

There are many asthma camps located in pollen-free areas which have a resident physician and which will keep a child all summer so that his return home coincides with the end of the allergy season. While at camp, the child must have an identification card containing his name, his phone number, his address, the name and phone number of his doctor, his blood type, his Rh factor, a list of his allergens, the dates of his immunizations, and an emergency kit to use for insect and bee stings. If he has eczema as well, he should avoid sweating (by controlling physical exercise) and excessive exposure to sunlight. He should swim in the ocean, but not in chlorinated pools. His desensitization program should continue while he is at camp.

The school of the asthmatic child should be an allergy-free place in which he may develop his personality, increase his knowledge, and learn to accept his shortcomings. While going to school in winter, he must be properly dressed, not with coarse woolen clothes, but with soft woolens* or synthetics, all of which must be taken out of storage and aired a few days before wearing. On cold days, he must wear a mask while in the street to avoid breathing frigid air. If riding a bus, he should sit near the driver where the fumes are less prevalent. In class, he should not erase blackboards or do cleaning chores that stir up dust or be near flowers, pets, or plants. His lunch should be prepared at home so he may avoid the foods to which he is allergic. (A list of those foods should be kept with him and in the cafeteria.)

---

*Unfortunately, most woolens are dyed, and since some children are allergic to dyes, the parent should watch carefully when a new garment is worn.

5

Desensitization—

ALSO KNOWN AS HYPOSENSITIZATION AND IMMUNOTHERAPY

Desensitization against allergy consists of a series of injections of small amounts of allergens administered at weekly intervals in increasing doses to diminish sensitivity. Once a maximum tolerated dose is reached after about four or five months, the injections are slowly spaced out until they are given at monthly intervals. If the child's symptoms disappear for a period of two years, he may stop his desensitization treatment.

Methods Used in Desensitization

There are three methods a doctor may use in desensitizing a patient:

Coseasonal method: starts injections during the season of the allergen.

Preseasonal method: starts injections three months before the onset of the season of the allergen. Dosage increases are made if an injection is well tolerated within a period of seven days of the preceding injection. If more than ten days pass between one injection and another, the dosage of the second injection must be reduced in proportion to the period of time that has elapsed. (The main reason for postponing an injection is serious illness. Minor colds and slight wheezes are not reasons for missing injections.)

Perennial method: Gives injections throughout the whole year and not merely in the weeks preceding the allergy season. This is the type of desensitization used by the majority of allergists. At the beginning of September, the first injection is given, followed in two weeks by another. A third injection is given three weeks later, and the fourth and subsequent injections are given at four-week intervals throughout the winter. Before the beginning of the next season, injections are resumed at weekly intervals.

Solutions Used in Desensitization

1. Aqueous extracts provide relief from the symptoms of inhalant allergy for about 80 percent of the patients properly treated.

2. Oily extracts (or the "one-shot" method) have been stopped by the Food and Drug Administration.

3. Allpyral allergens are absorbed slowly and cause fewer side effects than aqueous extracts; however, a final verdict on their use is still to come.

4. Detoxified extracts or allergoids are still experimental.

5. Oral desensitization is of questionable value.

Reactions to Desensitization

Desensitizing injections may cause a local reaction or a generalized one. The local reaction is a redness and soreness in the place of the injection. It is to be managed with ice packs and antihistamines. If the redness is as large as a fifty-cent piece, the same dose of allergen has to be repeated the following week. A generalized reaction may consist of hives, tightness in the chest, running of the nose, asthma, cyanosis, flushing, perspiration, nausea, vomiting, dizziness, or fainting. Should it occur, a tourniquet must be tied above the place of the injection; ⅓ cc. of adrenalin should be injected subcutaneously and repeated in half an hour if necessary. Hydrocortisone (1.25 mg.) should be given intramuscularly.

After a generalized reaction, the amount of allergen to be given the following week is to be reduced to one-half the previous dose. Generalized reactions in desensitization indicate that there is a need to decrease the dosage of the injection, but they are not an indication to stop the injections completely.

In exceptional circumstances, desensitization may be given at home by a parent trained by a physician. The parent should be sure to:

a. Keep the desensitization vials in the dark and in a refrigerator.
b. Keep a vial of adrenalin and one of hydrocortisone at hand.
c. Keep a disposable syringe with a ⅜-inch, 26-gauge needle ready for use.

The allergenic extract must be drawn in an allergy syringe, the excess air being pushed out. The injection site should be cleaned with alcohol, and the injection given in the arm. The piston should be pulled back to make sure there is no blood drawn into the syringe. Afterwards, the child must be kept quiet for twenty minutes.

Desensitization Results

Desensitization may fail because it was not accompanied by elimination of all the allergens to which the child is sensitive; the allergen injected was not selected on the basis of a history and skin tests; it did not follow a proper schedule (too much allergen injected reproduces the disease, while too little does not protect against it) ; a focus of infection sustaining the allergy was not eliminated by removing the tonsils and adenoids.

Helpful adjuncts to a desensitization program are a well-balanced diet, exercise, recreation, and rest. An allergic child should sleep ten to twelve hours a night, have a one- to two-hour nap in the afternoon, avoid fatigue, and have no rough or wild play. He should also avoid common colds, overexertion, and quick changes in temperature, as these disturb the allergic equilibrium by furnishing additional burdens to the system and allow existing allergies to become worse or develop more frequently.

Appendix

DRUGS USED IN ASTHMA (PATENTED)

Alupent
Aminodur Dura Tabs
Asbron
Brethine AB
Bricanyl Sulfate
Bronkotabs
Cromolyn Sodium marketed as:
  (a) Intal
  (b) Aarane
Duovent

Fleet Theophylline Rectal Enema (premeasured, prefilled, and prelubricated)
Isuprel Mistometer
Lufyllin GG
Marax
Metaprel
Quandrinal
Tedral Antiasthmatic
Tedral Expectorant
Vanceril

INSTITUTES FOR THE REHABILILATION OF CHRONIC ASTHMA

CALIFORNIA
Stanford Children's Convalescent Hospital
520 Willow Rd.
Palo Alto (94304)

Sunair Home for Asthmatic Children
775 McGroarty Ave.
Tujunga (91042)

COLORADO
National Jewish Hospital
3800 East Colfax Ave.
Denver (80206)

Children's Asthma Research Institute and Hospital
3401 West 19th Ave.
Denver (80204)

DISTRICT OF COLUMBIA
Hospital for Sick Children
1731 Bunker Hill Road NE
Washington (20017)

FLORIDA
Asthmatic Children's Foundation
Residential Treatment Center
1800 Northeast 168th St.
North Miami Beach (33162)

ILLINOIS
LaRabida Children's Hospital
Research Center
65th At Lake Michigan
Chicago (60649)

KENTUCKY
Cardinal Hiss Convalescent Hospital
2050 Versailles Rd.
Lexington (40504)

MARYLAND
Happy Hills Hospital Incorporated
1708 West Rogers Ave.
Baltimore (21209)

MASSACHUSETTS
Lakeville Hospital Asthma Rehabilitation Unit
Lakeville (02346)

MICHIGAN
Mary Free Bed Hospital & Rehabilitation Center
920 Cherry St. SE
Grand Rapids (49506)

NEW JERSEY
Children's Seashore House
4100 Atlantic Ave.
Atlantic City (08401)

Betty Bacharach Home for Afflicted Children
24th and Atlantic Ave.
Longport (08403)

NEW YORK
St. Mary's Hospital for Children
20-01 126th St.
Bayside (11360)

New York Infirmary
321 E. 15th St.
New York City (10003)

Blythedale Children's Hospital
Valhalla (10595)

OHIO
Convalescent Hospital for Children
119 Wellington Pl.
Cincinnati (45219)

Health Hill Hospital for Children
Cleveland (44104)

OKLAHOMA
Children's Convalescent Hospital
P.O. Box 888
Oklahoma City

PENNSYLVANIA
Children's Heart Hospital
Conshohocken Rd.
Philadelphia (19131)

VERMONT
Caverly Child Health Center
Pittsford (05763)

CANADA
Queen Alexandra Solarium for Crippled Children
British Columbia

Ontario Crippled Children's Center
350 Rumsey Road
Ontario (17)

DRUGS USED IN HAYFEVER

Nasal Vasoconstrictors
(Solutions and Sprays)

Neo-Synephrine   Allerest Nasal Spray
Alcon-Efrin   Afrin Nasal Spray

Privine   Eye Drops:
Tyzine   Prefrin
Otrivin   Vasocon
Turbinaire Decadron   Visine
Coricidin Nasal Mist

Representative Antihistamines Used in the Treatment of Allergic Rhinitis

Antihistamines are generally classified on the basis of chemical structure. Because of similar structures, a member of one class exhibits pharmacological properties similar to those of the other members of that class.

Class I Ethanolamines

PRODUCT	CHARACTERISTIC PROPERTIES OF THE CLASS
Benadryl	As a group have marked
Clistin	sedative effects. Low
Hydrylline	incidence of gastroin-
Naldecon	testinal effects. Dura-
Rondec	tion of action, three
Sinubid	to four hours.
Sinutab	

Class II Ethylenediamines

Co-Pyronil	Lower incidence of sedation than Class I.
Histadyl	Higher incidence of gastrointestinal effects than Class I.
Rynatan	Duration of action, three to six hours.

Class III Alkylamines

Actidil	
Actifed	Not especially liable to
Chlortrimeton	produce drowsiness.
Coricidin	Central nervous system

Coryban
Co-Tylenol
Covanamine
Covangesic
Deconamine
Demazine
Dimetapp
Disomer
Dor-C
Drixoral
Duadocin
Histaspan
Hycomine
Metreton
Naldecon
Napril
Novahistine
Ornade
Polaramine
Quelidrine
Robitussin A-C
Rynatan
Teldrin
Triaminic
Trisulfaminic
Tussagesic
Tussaminic
Tuss-Organidin
Ursinus
Ventilade

stimulation more common side effect.

Duration of action usually six hours, but some members act for eight to twelve hours.

Class IV Piperazines

Tacaryl

Used primarily to counter motion sickness.

Low incidence of drowsiness.

Duration of action, four to six hours.

Class V Phenothiazines

Phenergan
Used mainly as major tranquilizer in psychological disorders.

Side effects include jaundice, agranulocytosis, bizarre neurological syndromes.

Duration of action, twelve to twenty-four hours.

Camps for Allergic Children

CALIFORNIA
Allergy Foundation of Northern California
Santa Cruz Mountains

KENTUCKY
Camp Weasel
Lexington

MINNESOTA
Camp Sdikrepus
Minneapolis

NEW YORK
Camp Massawixie
Adirondack Mountains

Wagon Road Camp
Chappaqua

WASHINGTON
Children's Orthopedic Hospital and Medical Center
    Camp
Seattle

WEST VIRGINIA
Bronco Junction
Red House

A GUIDE TO WHEN—WHERE —WHICH POLLEN

For purposes of pollen evaluation, the United States can arbitrarily be divided into ten areas.

    a. Alaska and Hawaii: These states are free from allergy-producing pollen throughout the year.

    b. Northeastern United States (Maine, New Hampshire, Vermont, New York, Massachusetts, Connecticut, Rhode Island, Pennsylvania, West Virginia, Delaware, and Maryland): Trees pollinate between February and May, although an occasional tree might pollinate in June. Grasses pollinate during May, June, and, occasionally, July. Weeds pollinate during the summer months, with ragweed most consistently occurring from mid-August to the first frost.

    c. South Atlantic states (Virginia, North Carolina, South Carolina, Georgia, and Florida): Trees pollinate from mid-January to mid-May. Grasses pollinate from April until September. Weeds pollinate during the month of July and from mid-August to the first frost.

    d. Mid-Southern and Gulf Area states (Tennessee, Alabama, Mississippi, Arkansas, Louisiana, and part of Texas): Trees pollinate from January through May. Grasses pollinate from May through September. Weeds pollinate from July to October.

e. States in the Great Lakes Area (Michigan, Ohio, Wisconsin, Illinois, Indiana, and Kentucky) : Trees pollinate during March and April. Grasses pollinate primarily during June and July. Weeds pollinate from June through September.

f. Middle Western states (Minnesota, Iowa, Missouri, Kansas, Nebraska, South Dakota, and North Dakota) : Trees pollinate primarily between April and May. Grasses pollinate during June through September. Weeds pollinate from July to September.

g. Great Plains states (parts of Iowa, Nebraska, the Dakotas, Kansas, and Minnesota) : Trees pollinate primarily in April and May. Grasses pollinate in June and July. Weeds pollinate in August and September.

h. Rocky Mountain states (Montana, Idaho, Wyoming, Colorado, and Utah) : Trees pollinate primarily in April and May. Grasses pollinate in June, July, and August. Weeds pollinate in August and September.

i. Northwestern states (Washington, Oregon, Nevada, and northern California) : Trees pollinate from March through April. Grasses pollinate from May through August. Weeds pollinate from August through October.

j. Southwestern states (New Mexico, Arizona, southern California, Oklahoma, and parts of Texas) : Trees pollinate from March through May. Grasses pollinate during the summer. Weeds pollinate during both summer and fall.

Hayfever Holiday

For ragweed sufferers in the United States who take their vacations during the ragweed season, and particularly for those with severe ragweed asthma, authentic advice as to the comparative aerial ragweed pollen pollution in various parts of the country is of the greatest importance.

We have found that the data compiled by Oren C. Durham for the pollen and mold committee of the American Academy of Allergy are the most authentic. We reproduce this information here in full.

The Ragweed Pollen Index

The exact index figures are based on factors which directly affect individual seasonal pollen exposure: length of season, maximum aerial concentration of pollen on any one day, and the accumulated annual total pollen catch on one square centimeter of horizontally exposed, oiled test-slide area throughout the season. Thus the pollen index is not just a pollen count, but a statistical approximation of the degree of effective exposure to ragweed pollen in each location studied.

Explanation of Symbols and Terms

Excellent: This category includes communities with perfect or nearly perfect ragweed pollen records.

Good: This category includes communities with somewhat more pollen contamination than the average count of those in the above designation, but it is unlikely that anyone will experience severe hayfever symptoms from the amounts to be encountered in any of these places.

Fairly good: In this category are communities where most ragweed victims will experience an adequate degree of relief during the ragweed season.

Not recommended: In this category one will find extremely high concentrations.

Ragweed Pollen Refuges in the U.S.A. and Its Island Territories

ALABAMA. The gulf coast at Foley, good; fairly good at Mobile. Field surveys throughout the remainder of the state reveal wide distribution of ragweeds in waste places and on farms. Birmingham has a very poor record.

ALASKA. No ragweed pollen was found as a result of atmospheric tests made for one season in three places, namely, Nome, Fairbanks, and Juneau.

ARIZONA. Excellent rating for the north and south rims of Grand Canyon. During the fall season in Phoenix, conditions are excellent, but there is a spring ragweed season of at least moderate consequence. Our best information for the Tucson area gives it a rating of good for both spring and fall. For other communities in the state, there are no atmospheric data.

ARKANSAS. The average exposure to ragweed pollen throughout the state is doubtless very heavy. No refuge areas are known.

CALIFORNIA. Excellent: Lassen Volcanic National Park, Sequoia National Park, Oakland, Sacramento, San Francisco, Monterey, Yountville, Yosemite National Park, Los An-

geles, Pasadena, El Centro, Escondido, San
Diego, Tujunga. Good: Alpine, Arcata, Santa
Barbara.

While air sampling has not been done in the
great central valley, it is unlikely that any
community there or elsewhere in the state will
be found to have an appreciable degree of
ragweed pollen pollution.

COLORADO. Excellent: Rocky Mountain
National Park at Estes Park and Grand Lake,
Mesa Verde National Park, Glenwood Springs,
the crest of Pikes Peak.

Colorado Springs has a good rating, although formerly this city's record was not so
good. Ragweeds are not common on the west of
the slope. Sagebrush is likely to be encountered in this area. Close exposure should be
avoided by ragweed-sensitive persons.

Denver and the eastern third of the state
constitutes an area of moderate to heavy
ragweed exposure.

CONNECTICUT. Atmospheric studies have
been made in eight cities. No refuge areas are
known.

DELAWARE. Field studies show ragweed
to be abundant throughout. Nearest atmospheric studies are those made at Philadelphia
and Baltimore. No refuge areas are known.

DISTRICT OF COLUMBIA and adjacent
areas of Maryland show heavy ragweed pollen
incidence.

FLORIDA. Excellent: Santa Rosa Island,
Key West, Fort Myers, Miami Beach, Coral
Gables, Miami, Sunnyside Beach (Panama
City). Good: Daytona Beach, Orlando, Se-
bring, Bradenton, Everglades National Park,
St. Petersburg, Fort Pierce, Live Oak, West

Palm Beach. Fairly good: Fort Lauderdale (Beach), Jacksonville, Tallahassee, Tampa, Clearwater, Pensacola. Not recommended: Ocala, Gainesville, Melbourne, Panama City.

The beaches of Florida are most uniformly desirable; inland areas often are not so good.

GEORGIA. Valdosta (only one season), fairly good. Central and northern Georgia and the coastal area, as judged by tests at Atlanta and Saint Simons Island and as checked by widely scattered field surveys, have moderately heavy exposure.

HAWAII. No significant amounts of any kind of ragweed have been found anywhere on the larger islands except in the area between Scofield Barracks and Pearl Harbor on Oahu. Honolulu is probably ragweed-pollen-free on account of prevailing northeast tradewinds. No daily atmospheric tests have ever been reported.

IDAHO. Excellent: Sun Valley, Moscow. Good: Boise, Pocatello.

All mountainous areas are excellent, but exposure to sagebrush pollen is possible throughout most of the state. Close contact with sagebrush should be strictly avoided.

ILLINOIS. No refuge area. Heavy records in seventeen cities and towns.

INDIANA. No refuge area. Heavy records in seven cities and towns.

IOWA. No refuge area. Heavy records in six cities and towns.

KANSAS. No refuge area. Atmospheric ragweed pollen incidence diminishes westwardly.

KENTUCKY. No refuge areas are known,

but are barely possible in the Cumberland Mountains.

LOUISIANA. Heavy atmospheric pollution at New Orleans. Air sampling has been carried on only at New Orleans and at Vicksburg, Mississippi, across the river from Tallulah, Louisiana.

MAINE. Excellent: St. Francis, Greenville Junction, Millinocket, Presque Isle, Macwahoc, Quoddy Head, New Portland, Newagen, Enfield, Deblois, Belfast, Allagash, Grand Lake Stream, Bethel, Eagle Lake, Lincoln, Oquossoc, Speckle Mountain, Upper Dam. Good: Houlton, Newport, Jackman, Machias, Bar Harbor, Boothbay Harbor. Fairly good: Eastport, Rockland, Southport, York, Augusta, Camden, Rangeley, North Augusta, Orono. Not recommended: Stonington, Polant Spring, Auburn, Alfred, Portland, Kineo.

MARYLAND. No refuge area is known. No atmospheric studies have been made in the mountainous parts of western Maryland.

MASSACHUSETTS. Good: Annisquam, East Gloucester, West Gloucester, Magnolia, Rockport, Nantucket Island. Not recommended: Winchester, Boston, Northampton, Amherst, Newton Center.

This is the state, and Boston the chief city, from which ragweed hayfever victims first fled to the mountains and rocky coastal areas of New Hampshire and Maine some 100 years ago. Even so, ragweed pollen is much less abundant in the air of Boston than in many of the larger cities of the northeastern United States. Of the fourteen communities tested, none offers excellent refuge conditions. Neither the Berkshires nor Cape Cod has received attention. Weed destruction seems to be effective on Nantucket Island. Otherwise, ragweeds take over all waste areas.

MICHIGAN. Excellent: Isle Royale National Park. Good: Sault Sainte Marie, Copper Harbor. Fairly good: Houghton.

Fifty years ago much of the area of northern Michigan was doubtless entirely free from ragweeds and ragweed pollen, but sampling done in fifty-seven systematically selected communities during the past twenty-five years has shown that no effective refuges remain in the lower peninsula and that those of the northern peninsula are few, as listed above. The following list does not include any city of the lower peninsula. Those listed at the beginning are much better than those toward the end and might be suitable for persons with moderate sensitivity.

Not recommended (upper peninsula only): Saint Ignace, Blaney, Munising, Ironwood, Mackinac Island, Newberry, Powers, Menominee, Encanaba.

MINNESOTA. Fairly good: Tower, Virginia. Other places as good as or better than Tower and Virginia could probably be found in other parts of Arrowhead County (northeastern corner of the state). The state has been inadequately covered. Not recommended: Duluth, Rochester, Minneapolis, Winona, Moorhead.

MISSISSIPPI. Biloxi, on the coast, is fairly good. Field studies reveal an abundance of ragweed on farms throughout, so, except for the immediate coast, no refuge areas are likely to be found.

MISSOURI. No refuge areas.

MONTANA. Excellent: Glacier National Park at Belton and Many Glacier, West Yellowstone. Good: Miles City.

Judging by the excellent records for more than twenty cities and towns in the adjacent parts of Alberta and Saskatchewan and at Yellowstone National Park, most of Montana is practically free of ragweeds.

Very meager data and no recent studies are available for this state. Sagebrush is widely distributed and should be avoided by persons known to be ragweed-sensitive.

NEBRASKA. No refuge areas, but considerably less ragweed is found in the western third of the state than in the eastern part.

NEVADA. Very meager data, and no recent air sampling. Ragweeds are rare along the principal highways. Reno is excellent, and Lake Mead is excellent in the fall, and good in the spring ragweed season. Sagebrush is a possible factor.

NEW HAMPSHIRE. Excellent: Moosilauke, Pawtackaway, Errol, Lancaster, Carroll, Laconia, Colebrook, Blue Job Mountains, Derry, Groveton, Lincoln, Pittsburg, Warren, Whitefield. Good: Bath, Conway, Dixville, Littleton, North Conway, Ossipee, Hampton, Plymouth, Bethlehem, Crotched Mountain, Dover, Franklin, New Ipswich, Manchester, Weirs. Not recommended: Hinsdale, Charlestown, Rye, Rochester, Lebanon, Jeremy, Exeter, Peterborough, Nashua.

NEW JERSEY. No refuge areas are known. Those places along the northern shore where relief is sometimes found are subject to high counts when the wind blows from the west. Studies have been made in twenty-nine cities.

NEW MEXICO. Very meager atmospheric data. Ragweeds are probably comparatively rare throughout the state. Roswell is good, and Albuquerque fairly good.

NEW YORK. The reports on Long Island have produced variable records. Fire Island at Ocean Beach is sometimes fairly good, and Montauk likewise is fairly good. No other records are available for the Island, except in Brooklyn, which is not recommended.

Excellent: Adirondack Mountain area, Keene Valley. Fairly good: Big Moose, Chilson, Indian Lake, Long Lake, McColloms, Raquette Lake, Paul Smiths, Redford, Wanakena, Chateaugay Lake, Inlet, Sabatiis, Schroon Lake (Severance), Tupper, Newcomb, Owl's Head, Lake Placid, McKeever. Good: The Catskill Mountain area, Big Indian, Haines Falls, Pine Hill. Fairly good: Fleischmanns.

Studies have been made in eighty-five communities, including all of the larger cities, none of which can be recommended.

NORTH CAROLINA. No refuge areas are known, but air tests at Newfound Gap, Tennessee, on the crest of the Great Smoky Mountains, prove the immediate area to be good. It is likely that there are other places equally good at similar or higher elevations in North Carolina. (There are no accommodations at Newfound Gap in the National Park.) There are records of heavy concentration of ragweed pollen for four of the large cities of the state.

NORTH DAKOTA. No atmospheric data are available except in the narrow Red River

Valley at Fargo. No refuge areas are known, but conditions are likely to be very similar in the southern half of the state as in South Dakota. Judging from data from adjacent areas in Canada, there might be some good places found along the north edge of the state.

OHIO. No refuge areas. Adequate sampling has been done in seven large cities.

OREGON. No atmospheric studies have been made in eastern Oregon except at Milton-Freewater, which is good.

Excellent: Coquille, Corvallis, Eugene, Crater Lake National Park, Portland, Turner.

PENNSYLVANIA. No refuge areas are known. Claims for mountain resorts have never been proved. Sampling has been carried on in ten large cities for many years.

PUERTO RICO. No atmospheric studies have ever been reported, but recent careful field examination failed to disclose any ragweeds on the island.

RHODE ISLAND. No refuge areas.

SOUTH CAROLINA. No refuge areas are known, but our data are very meager. Nothing recent.

SOUTH DAKOTA. There are no refuge areas better than fairly good. Fairly good: Rapid City, Mobridge.

TENNESSEE. No refuge areas are known. Along the crest of the Great Smoky Mountains at Newfound Gap, conditions were found to be good. There are no accommodations at this point, but there might be places with similar conditions at similar or higher elevations.

TEXAS. From among the ten communities where studies have been made, Big Spring is the only one which has a rating of good. Most of Texas is badly infested with ragweeds. However, they diminish considerably toward the western corner of the state, as for example in El Paso.

UTAH. Excellent: Zion National Park, Bryce Canyon National Park.

Vernal in the extreme northeast corner of the state and Hurricane in the extreme southwest corner of the state are fairly good. The average for metropolitan Salt Lake City is also fairly good, except for the Canyon Rim area.

VERMONT. Very meager data. Conditions on the east side of the state are probably comparable to adjacent areas of New Hampshire. Heavy atmospheric contamination is found in the upper Lake Champlain area.

VIRGINIA. No excellent or good refuges are known.

VIRGIN ISLANDS. Excellent: The island of St. John (Virgin Islands National Park), the island of St. Thomas.

WASHINGTON. Excellent: Seattle-Tacoma Airport, Mt. Rainier National Park (Longmire, White River, Paradise Valley), Seattle, Olympic National Park, Spokane, Yakima. Good: Walla Walla.

Except for the badly ragweed-contaminated orchards in the immediate vicinity of Wenatchee, all but one place among the ten tested in the state are excellent or good.

WEST VIRGINIA. No refuge areas are known.

WISCONSIN. No refuge areas are known, but no adequate investigation has been made in the vast lake region of the northern part of the state.

WYOMING. Excellent: Grand Teton National Park, Yellowstone National Park. Not recommended: Lander.

Very meager data except at the national parks.

Ragweed Pollen Refuges in Canada

ALBERTA. With atmospheric tests in fourteen communities, we have the following to report. Excellent: Banff, Beaver Lodge, Edmonton, Jasper, Vermilion, Lake Louise, Cypess Hill, Waterton Lakes Park, Calgary, Coleman, Manyberries, Drumheller, Lethbridge. Fairly good: Medicine Hat. Sagebrush pollen is a possible irritant to ragweed sufferers in those parts of Alberta which have been covered by the surveys.

BRITISH COLUMBIA. Meager data. Excellent: Summerland, Saanichton, Victoria.

MANITOBA. Excellent: The Pas, Riding Mountain National Park, Russell, Brandon. Good: Douphin. Fairly good: Pierson, Winnipeg. Sagebrush pollen is a possible irritant to ragweed sufferers in those parts of Manitoba which have been covered by the surveys.

NEW BRUNSWICK. Excellent: Campbellton, Bathurst, Richibucto, Newcastle-Chatam, Dalhousie, Fredericton, Woodstock, Doaktown, McAdam, Shediac Cape, St. John, Grand Manan, Edmundston, Perth-Andover, St. George, Welsford, St. Andrews, St. Stephan, Chipman, Moncton, Sackville, Tracadie. Good: Sussex, Haslam Farm (Fundy National Park), Lakeview, Jemseg, Waterside (Fundy National Park). Fairly good: Pointe-du-Chêne, Gagetown. No high concentrations were found at any place.

NEWFOUNDLAND. Only two communities

on the island have been studied: Corner Brook and St. John's, both excellent.

NOVA SCOTIA. Excellent: Truro, Middle West Pubnico, Cape Breton Highlands National Park, Chester, Antigonish, Baddeck, Ingonish Island. Good: Meteghan, Digby, Yarmouth, Kentville. No other studies have been reported.

ONTARIO. Systemic atmospheric pollen research has been carried on in Ontario since 1928, gradually increasing in volume until records are now available for at least one season in seventy communities. For some communities there are now continuous annual records for more than thirty years. The well-populated area of southern Ontario from Windsor to Cornwall is about as heavily contaminated with ragweed as are the adjacent areas of the U.S.A. But farther northward and northwestward, in areas of less intensive cultivation or none at all, air pollution drops rapidly to insignificant levels.

Excellent: Timmins, Fort William, New Liskeard, Kapuskasing, Port Arthur, Fort Francis, Barry's Bay, Black Sturgeon Lake, Chalk River, Cochrane, South River, Haliburton. Good: Blind River, Mattawa, Temegami, Lake Joseph, Magnetawan, Rosseau, Sudbury, Espanola, Muskata Falls, Tobermory. Fairly good: Cedar Lake, Dorset, Pembroke, Renfrew, Sault Sainte Marie, Honey Harbor, Bancroft, Kenora, Mindemoya (Manitoulin Island), North Bay, Westport, Port Carling.

Places not recommended, at least for severe cases, are listed here in order of their degree of air pollution from the least to greatest: Huntsville, Smith Falls, Algonquin Park, Georgian Bay Islands National Park, Gravenhurst, Lion's Head, Ottawa, Parry Sound, Madoc, Wiarton, Cornwall, Kincardine, Belleville, Peterborough, Picton, St. Lawrence Islands National Park, Dondon, Mallorytown, Toronto and metropolitan area, Windsor, Hamilton.

PRINCE EDWARD ISLAND. Excellent: Cavendish, Montague, Souris, Summerside, Tignish, Charlottetown, O'Leary. Good: Prince Edward National Park. No other studies have been reported.

QUEBEC. Excellent: Chandler, Iles-de-la-Madeleine, Matapédia, Mont-Albort Gaspésie, Gaspé, Grande-Rivière, Mont-Joli, Father Point, Carleton, Charlesbourg, Jonquière (Chicoutimi), Lennoxville, Sainte-Lambert. Fairly good: Sainte-Jovite, Nominingue, Ste. Anne-de-la-Pocatire, Ste. Agathe, Lac-des-Seize Illes, Lac-des-Plages, Mont-Laurier, Mont Tremblant, Rimouski, Rivière-du-Loup. In the southwest tip of the province, adjacent to New York and New Hampshire, air contamination is bad. North of the Ottawa and St. Lawrence River and in the Gaspé country, conditions are good to excellent.

SASKATCHEWAN. Excellent: Prince Albert National Park, Nelford, Prince Albert, Scott, Regina, Saskatoon, Swift Current.

Ragweed Pollen Refuges on Bermuda

Atmospheric tests have been made only at Hamilton where no ragweed pollen was detected.

Ragweed Pollen Refuges in Mexico

Good: Mexico City, Tampico, Torreon. Not recommended: Ciudad Juàrez, Matamorors.

Slender false ragweed and western ragweed are found in small amounts in all states as far south as Mexico City. Our best information is that ragweed pollen concentrations are very low in most parts and absent in the southern states.

PROPRIETARY DRUGS CONTAINING ASPIRIN

Acetidine	Coricidin	Midol
Alka-Seltzer	Dristan	Pepto-Bismol
Anacin	Ecotrin	Persistin
Anahist	Empirin	Stanback
APC	Compound	Theracin
Aspergum	Excedrin	Triaminicin
BC	Inhiston	Trigesic
Bromo-Quinine	Measurin	Vanquish
Bromo-seltzer		
Bufferin		

Aspirin Substitutes

Acetaminophen is sold as Liquiprin, Tempra, Tylenol, and Valadol.

DRUGS AND AGENTS USED IN ECZEMA

Tranquilizers—Antihistamines Used To Control the Itch in Eczema
Atarax
Vistaril

Cleansing Agents

Lowila Cake, Aveeno Bar, Petrophyllic Soap, Cetaphil Lotion, Neutrogena Soaps, Oilatum Soap, Polytar Soap, Alpha Keri Soap, Lubriderm Soap.

Antipruritic Baths
Aveeno Colloidal Oatmeal (Argo, Linit, or Niagra).

Vinyl Gloves for Contact Eczema
These may be obtained in a thin vinyl or a utility household heavy-duty vinyl from Bard-Parker and Co., a division of the Becton-Dickinson Co., Rutherford, New Jersey; and from Arbrook, Inc., Arlington, Texas.

Silicone-Based Ointments for Contact Eczema
Covicone Cream, Silicote Ointment (Cream or Spray), Silon Spray, Kerodex Cream.

Topical Corticosteroids
These represent a major advance in the local treatment of eczema and should be used according to their specifications.

Antibiotic Ointments and Creams Used in Infected Eczema

TRADE NAME	MARKETED AS	THERAPEUTIC ACTION
Neosporin	Ointment	Antibacterial
	Cream	Antibacterial
Polysporin	Ointment	Antibacterial
Garamycin	Ointment	Anticandidal activity
	Cream	Anticandidal activity
Chloromycetin	Ointment	Anticandidal activity

	Cream	Anticandidal activity
Mycolog	Ointment	Anticandidal activity
	Cream	Anticandidal activity

Suncreening Agents Used To Protect The Skin in Eczema

Foremost among sunscreening agents are the preparations based on paraminobenzoic acid or PABA, marketed under these different names: Sundare Clear Lotion (Texas), Sunswept Cream (Texas), Sunstick (Texas), A-Fil Cream (Texas), Solbar Lotion (Person & Covey), UVAL Lotion (Dome), R.V.P. Ointment (Elder), R.V. Pellent Ointment (Elder), R.V. Racque Ointment (Elder), R.V. Plus Ointment (Elder), R.V. Paba Lipstick (Elder), Presun Lotion (Westwood), Eclipse Sunscreen Lotion (G.S. Herbert,) Pabafilm Gel (Owen), Pabanol Lotion (Elder), Pabagel Sunscreen Gel (Owen).

Packs Used for Acutely Inflamed Eczema

Packs may be prepared from the following:

Domeboro Powder Packets, Domeboro Effervescent Tablets (Dome)

Boro-Sol (Doak Pharmacal Corporation)

Bluboro Powder (Derm Arts Laboratories)

Aveeno Colloidal Oatmeal (Cooper Laboratories)

Burrow's Solution

Potassium Permanganate Tablets

VACCINES USED FOR CHILDREN

The initials used for these vaccines are

DPT—Diptheria, pertussis (whopping cough), and tetanus

M—Measles

Mu—Mumps

TOPV— Trivalent oral polio vaccine

R—Rubella

MMR—Measles, Mumps, Rubella

Td—Diptheria and tetanus

T—Tetanus

Simultaneous Administration

Simultaneous administration of combined measles/mumps/rubella (or measles/rubella) vaccine with Trivalent oral polio vaccine is possible.

Interruption of Immunization Schedule

A delay between scheduled immunizations does not interfere with final immunity. It does not necessitate starting the series over again, regardless of the interval elapsed. Simply pick up the schedule where left off.

Contraindications

DPT—Use with caution if there is: (a) a history of adverse reaction (fractionated doses of DPT may be given); (b) any febrile illness; (c) steroid therapy.

Oral polio*—Not routinely recommended for those: (a) over eighteen years of age; (b) with moderate or severe febrile illness; (c)

*Taken by mouth; not injected.

with persistent vomiting or diarrhea; (d) with any altered immune state.

Measles, Mumps, Rubella—Whether these vaccines are given individually, simultaneously, or in combined form, the following contraindications apply: (a) moderate to severe febrile illness; (b) leukemia or other malignancy; (c) steroids or other immunologic depressant; (d) immune serum globulin administered in previous six weeks; (e) egg sensitivity (if vaccine is prepared in egg); (f) active, untreated tuberculosis (tuberculin skin test can be given on the same day that the vaccine is given—if not given on the same day, TB skin test should be delayed for six weeks following a measles, rubella, or mumps immunization; (g) any other altered immune state.

SOURCES OF SUPPLIES AND AIDS

A few sources of products which may be useful for allergy patients are listed here. Lists are by no means complete and should only be considered as possible suggestions, not specific endorsements.

For general information, write to the Allergy Foundation of America, 801 Second Avenue, New York, N.Y. 10017.

Dust Masks and Heated Masks

These masks may be helpful when cleaning dusty areas, painting, or even cutting grass. Flex-A-Lite All-Purpose Mask, which has replaceable micro-foam filters, costs about $2.50

and is available from Allergen-Proof Encasings, Inc., 1450 E. 363rd St., Eastlake, Ohio 44094. Dustfoe 66 Respiratory Mask costs about $5.00 and is a quality product. It can be obtained from Mine Safety Appliance Co., 201 North Braddock Avenue, Pittsburgh, Pennsylvania 15208. In an emergency, use any "painter's mask" which can be bought in paint stores.

A special mask heated by an electric battery made for this purpose is the Weather Guard Mask made by Carman Commodities Corporation, 2900 West Peterson Ave., Chicago, Illinois 60645.

Another useful mask made to filter urban air without reducing its oxygen content is manufactured by Hine Safety Appliances and marketed by Survival Associates. It is to be worn by children with respiratory problems during periods of heavy air pollution to guard them against lung irritation and infection.

Humidity Gauges
Two brand names are Skuttle Hygrometer, and the Taylor Water Humidiguide.

Mold Preventatives
Captan is the trade name of a mold preventative which may be obtained at most garden-supply stores or nurseries. For more information write to the U.S. Department of Agriculture, Washington, D.C. Impregon may be obtained from Fleming and Company, 9730 Reavis Park Drive, St. Louis, Missouri 63123.

For the nearest distributor of Paraformaldehyde, write to J.T. Baker Chemical Co., Execu-
tive Offices and Plant, Phillipsburg, New
Jersey 08865.

Stinging-Insect Kits
Hollister-Stier Laboratories: Downer's Grove,
Illinois; Spokane, Washington; Atlanta, Geor-
gia; Dallas, Texas; Burbank and Livermore,
California; Yeadon, Pennsylvania; Mississ-
aqua, and Ontario, Canada.

Disposable Allergy Syringes with Needles
Becton-Dickinson, Rutherford, New Jersey.

ALLERGY JOURNALS

The following journals carry articles dealing
exclusively with recent clinical and experimental developments in the field of allergy. Papers
of interest may also be found in many of the
journals of internal medicine, pediatrics, pul-
monary disease, dermatology, otolaryngology,
and immunology.

The Journal of Allergy, official organ of the
American Academy of Allergy, published
monthly by C.V. Mosby Co., 3207 Washington
Blvd., St. Louis, Missouri 63103.

Annals of Allergy, official journal of the
American College of Allergists, published
monthly at 2642 University Ave., St. Paul,
Minnesota 55114.

International Archives of Allergy and Ap-

plied Immunology, published monthly by S. Karger, Basel, Switzerland, and New York, New York.

Review of Allergy, containing abstracts and bibliography of current literature of allergy and allied fields, published monthly at 2642 University Ave., St. Paul, Minnesota 55114.

Acta Allergologica, official organ of the Northern Society of Allergology and of the European Academy of Allergology, published at irregular intervals (generally six or more issues per year) and Munksgaard, Prags Boulevard 47, Copenhagen S, Denmark.

NATIONAL HEALTH ORGANIZATIONS AND AGENCIES CONCERNED WITH PEDIATRIC ALLERGY

ALLERGY FOUNDATION OF AMERICA
801 Second Avenue
New York, New York

AMERICAN ACADEMY OF PEDIATRICS
1801 Hinman Avenue
Evanston, Illinois

AMERICAN PUBLIC HEALTH ASSOCIATION, INC.
1740 Broadway
New York, New York

AMERICAN SCHOOL HEALTH ASSOCIATION
515 East Main Street
Kent, Ohio

AMERICAN COLLEGE OF NUTRITION
American Nutrition Society

10651 West Pico Boulevard
Los Angeles, California

AMERICAN ASSOCIATION FOR REHABILITATION
THERAPY
12021 Joan Drive
Pittsburgh, Pennsylvania

NATIONAL ASSOCIATION OF RECREATIONAL THERA-
PISTS, INC.
Athens State Hospital
Athens, Ohio

BREATHING EXERCISES

The following exercises were taken from the American Academy of Pediatrics and can be used in this format with your child.

Do you know how to breathe? Sure you do . . . but do you know there is a *right* way and a *wrong* way to breathe?

Let me show you how you can learn the *right* way to breathe.

First, let's look at your chest to see how we breathe.

The way you start is

1. Lie down on the floor.

2. Bend your knees and keep your feet on the floor.

3. Put your arms at your sides.

Now . . . take a *deep* breath . . . and let it out . . . slowly. See what moves? Your chest and abdomen go up and down. Do it again . . . a few times.

Now try this. Put one hand on the top part of your chest . . . put your other hand on your abdomen . . . and breathe in through your nose.

Your *abdomen* should go *out* like a balloon. Your chest should not move.

Inhaling is using the *diaphragm*.

Try it again . . . as you pull air in through your *nose*, the hand on your chest is still . . . only the hand on your abdomen goes *up*. As you blow the air *out* through *pursed lips*, the hand on your abdomen goes *down* . . . the hand on your chest stays still.

Now let's practice *abdominal breathing*: Fold your hands on your abdomen . . . breathe in through your nose . . . see your abdomen get round like a ball? Do this ten times, making sure your chest remains still.

Now let's try the *most important* part of breathing, exhaling. Blow *all* the air out through your mouth, using pursed lips. Use the hand on your abdomen to help *press* all the air out.

Now your abdomen should be flat. Do this ten times, *slowly*.

Just for fun, put a *book* on your abdomen. See if you can make the book *fall off* as you take in air and make your abdomen round. Your abdomen should get *flat* again as you blow all the air out.

Remember to keep your chest still.

Here is another way.

Sit in a chair, nice and tall. Hold a book against your abdomen. Breathe in some air and let your abdomen *push out* against the book. Now, *push the book* hard against your abdomen.

Bend over . . . at the same time *blowing out* air. Do it the same way, ten times, *slowly*.

Try this the next time . . . and every time . . . you feel short of breath. Sit leaning forward with a straight back, your arms resting on your knees. Now, breathe in through your nose, then blow *all* the air out through your mouth slowly, keeping your chest still. Breathing this way will make you feel better and less tired.

If the exercises make you *cough*, this is good—it will help to dislodge any sputum.

Try lying over the side of the bed for ten to fifteen minutes to *drain out* the sputum. We can help you cough it out by clapping gently on your back. You will feel much better every time you do this!

Can you walk with a book balanced on your head? You can keep a *good posture* by remembering to stand up straight with your shoulders relaxed. Don't forget to keep your back flat against the chair when sitting.

Now you know how to breathe. See if you can do it this way *all the time*, sitting, standing, running, playing, working, at home . . . at school . . . everywhere.

Let's keep a record. . . . Make an X each day you do your breathing exercises.

Sunday

Monday

Tuesday

Wednesday

Thursday

Friday

Saturday

READY-MADE ALLERGY-FREE FOODS

Nabisco Products That Do Not Contain Milk or Milk Products

Brazil nut cookies
Brownie thin wafers
Chipsters potato snacks
Chocolate chip snaps
Chocolate covered gra-
hams
Chocolate Pinwheels
cakes
Chocolate snaps
Cinnamon graham treats
Comet cones
Comet cups
Comet pilot cones
Cookie Break vanilla
flavored creme sand-
wich
Cookie Break vanilla
wafers
Cream of Wheat cereal—
instant mix'n eat,
quick, regular
Crown pilot crackers
Dairy wafers round
Dandy soup and oyster
crackers
Dromedary corn bread
mix
Dromedary corn muffin
mix
Dromedary dates
Dromedary gingerbread
mix
Family favorites pecan
drop cookies
French onion crackers
Gem soup and chili
crackers
Lemon jumble rings
Lemon snaps
Meal Mates sesame
bread wafers
Mister Salty pretzel
rings
Mister Salty 3-ring pret-
zels
Mister Salty veri-thin
pretzels
Mister Salty veri-thin
pretzel sticks
Nabisco graham cracker
crumbs
Nabisco graham crack-
ers
Nabisco iced fruit cook-
ies
Nabisco iced oatmeal
raisin cookies
Nabisco 100% bran

Nabisco pecan short-
bread cookies
Nabisco rice honeys
Nabisco spiced wafers
Old fashion ginger snaps
Oysterettes soup and
oyster crackers
Premium crackers, un-
salted tops
Premium saltine crack-
ers
Pretzelettes
Ritz crackers
Sociables crackers
Soup Mates tiny soup
crackers
Spoon Size shredded
wheat
Sugar Honey Maid gra-
ham crackers

Team flakes
Triangle Thins crackers
Triscuit wafers
Uneeda biscuit, unsalted
tops
Vanilla crumbs
Veri-Thin pretzel sticks
Waverly wafers
Wheat thins crackers
Zu-Zu ginger snaps

Nabisco Products That Do Not Contain Wheat

Cheese flavored Flings
curls
Chipsters potato snacks
Corn Diggers snacks
Dromedary dates
Dromedary fudge and
frosting mix
Dromedary pimientos
Korkers corn chips

Nabisco rice honeys
Nabisco salted peanuts
Shapies cheese flavored
dip delights
Shapies cheese flavored
shells
Snack Mate pasteurized
process cheese spreads

Nabisco Products That Do Not Contain Egg

Appeteasers tiny crack-
ers, crescent-roll-shap-
ed
Appeteasers tiny crack-
ers, ham tasting/
shaped

Appeteasers tiny onion
shaped/flavored
Bacon flavored thin
crackers

Bali Hai Hawaiian flavor creme sandwich

Barnum's Animal crackers

Biscos sugar wafers

Biscos waffles

Brazil nut cookies

Brown edge wafers

Brownie thin wafers

Brownie thin wafers vanilla flavored

Butter flavored thins crackers

Butter flavored sesame snack crackers

Cameo creme sandwich

Cheese cracker, small

Cheese cracker squares

Cheese flavored Flings curls

Cheese'n bacon flavored sandwich

Cheese Nips crackers

Cheese-on-rye sandwich

Cheese peanut butter sandwich variety pack

Cheese sandwich

Cheese Tid-Bits crackers

Chicken in a Biskit crackers

Chippers potato crackers

Chips Ahoy! chocolate chip cookies

Chipsters potato snacks

Chocolate chip cookies

Chocolate chip snacks

Chocolate covered grahams

Chocolate crumbs

Chocolate Pinwheels cakes

Chocolate snaps

Cinnamon graham treats

Cocoanut bars cookies

Comet pilot cones

Cookie Break assorted fudge creme sandwich

Cookie Break chocolate fudge creme sandwich

Cookie Break sugar wafers

Corn Diggers snack

Cowboys and Indians cookies

Cream of Wheat cereals, instant mix'n eat, quick, regular

Creme wafer sticks

Crown peanut bars

Crown pilot crackers

Dairy wafers, round

Dandy soup and oyster crackers

Doo Dads snacks

Dromedary banana nut roll

Dromedary chocolate nut roll

Dromedary cornbread mix

Dromedary corn muffin mix

Dromedary date nut roll

Dromedary fudge and frosting mix

Dromedary orange nut roll

Dromedary pimientos

Dromedary pound cake mix

Escort crackers

Family Favorites chocolate chip cookies

Family Favorites chocolate nut cookies

Family Favorites raisin buns cookies

French onion cracker

Fudge creme sandwich cookies

Gem soup and chili crackers

Graham cracker crumbs

Graham crackers

Ideal chocolate peanut logs

Hey Days caramel peanut logs

Lemon snaps

Mallowmars chocolate cakes

Malted milk peanut butter sandwich

Marshmallow puffs

Marshmallow Twirls

Meal Mates sesame bread wafers

Melody chocolate cookies

Minarets cakes

Mint sandwich cookies

Mister Salty pretzel rings

Mister Salty 3-ring pretzels

Mister Salty Veri-Thin pretzels

Mister Salty Veri-Thin pretzel sticks

Nabisco devil's food cakes

Nabisco fancy crest cakes

Nabisco iced fruit cookies

Nabisco iced oatmeal rasin cookies

Nabisco macaroon sandwich

Nabisco oatmeal cookies

Nabisco raisin fruit biscuit

Nabisco salted peanuts

Nabisco shredded wheat

Nabisco spiced wafers

Nabisco rice honeys

Oreo creme sandwich

O-So-Gud cheese peanut butter sandwich

Oysterettes soup and oyster crackers

Pantry grahams

Peanut butter & jelly tasting patties

Peanut creme patties

Peanut creme sticks

Premium crackers, unsalted tops

Premium saltine crackers

Pretzelettes

Ritz cheese crackers

Ritz crackers

Shapies cheese flavored dip delights

Shapies cheese flavored shells

Sip'n Chips cheese flavored snacks

Snack Mates pasteurized process cheese spreads

Sociables crackers
Soup Mates tiny soup crackers
Spoon-Size shredded wheat
Striped shortbread
Sugar Honey Maid graham crackers
Swiss'n ham flavored Flings curls
Team flakes
Toastettes toaster pastries
Triangle Thins crackers
Triscuit wafers
Twigs sesame/cheese flavored snack sticks
Uneeda biscuit, unsalted tops
Vanilla crumbs
Waverly wafers
Wheat Honey cereal
Wheat thins crackers
Zu-Zu ginger snaps

Heinz Baby Foods

The following allergy-free baby foods are manufactured by Heinz.

Corn-Free Junior Foods

FRUITS
Apples and Pears
Applesauce
Applesauce and Apricots
Peaches
Pears
Pears and Pineapple

VEGETABLES
Carrots
Green Beans
Sweet Potatoes

MEATS
Beef and Beef Broth
Chicken and Chicken Broth
Chicken Sticks
Lamb and Lamb Broth
Veal and Veal Broth

Corn-Free Instant Cereals

Barley   Oatmeal

High Protein   Rice

Corn-Free Strained Foods

FRUITS

Apples and Pears

Applesauce

Applesauce and Apri-
cots

Peaches

Pears

Pears and Pineapple

MEATS AND EGG YOLKS

Beef and Beef Broth

Chicken and Chicken
Broth

Egg Yolks

Ham and Ham Broth

Lamb and Lamb Broth

Liver and Liver Broth

Pork and Pork Broth

Turkey and Turkey
Broth

Veal and Veal Broth

BREAKFASTS

Mixed Cereal with
Apples and Bananas

Oatmeal with Apples
and Bananas

Rice Cereal with Apples
and Bananas

JUICES

Apple

Apple-Apricot

Apple-Cherry

Apple-Grape

Apple-Pineapple

Mixed Fruit

Apple-Prune

Orange

Orange-Apple-Banana

Orange-Pineapple

VEGETABLES

Beets

Carrots

Green Beans

Squash

Sweet Potatoes

Wheat-Free Junior Foods

FRUITS
Apples and Cranberries
  with Tapioca
Apples and Pears
Applesauce
Applesauce and Apricots
Apricots with Tapioca
Bananas and Pineapple
  with Tapioca
Cottage Cheese with
  Bananas
Peaches
Pears
Pears and Pineapple

MEATS
Beef and Beef Broth
Chicken and Chicken
  Broth
Chicken Sticks
Lamb and Lamb Broth
Meat Sticks
Veal and Veal Broth

DESSERTS
Custard Pudding
Fruit Dessert
Pineapple Orange
  Dessert
Tutti Frutti

HIGH MEAT DINNERS
Beef with Vegetables
  and Cereal
Chicken with Vegetables
Ham with Vegetables
Turkey with Vegetables
Veal with Vegetables

DINNER AND SOUPS
Chicken Soup
Vegetables and Bacon
Vegetables and Beef

VEGETABLES
Carrots
Creamed Corn
Creamed Peas
Green Beans
Mixed Vegetables
Sweet Potatoes

Wheat-Free Instant Cereals
Barley   Rice
Oatmeal

Wheat-Free Strained Foods

FRUITS

Apples and Cranberries
Apples and Pears
Applesauce
Apricots with Tapioca
Bananas and Pineapple
Bananas with Tapioca
Cottage Cheese with Bananas
Peaches
Pears
Pears and Pineapple
Plums with Tapioca
Prunes with Tapioca

JUICES

Apple
Apple-Apricot
Apple-Cherry
Apple-Grape
Apple-Pineapple
Apple-Prune
Mixed Fruit
Orange
Orange-Apple-Banana
Orange-Pineapple

MEATS AND EGG YOLKS

Beef and Beef Broth
Chicken and Chicken Broth
Egg Yolks
Ham and Ham Broth
Lamb and Lamb Broth
Liver and Liver Broth
Pork and Pork Broth
Turkey and Turkey Broth
Veal and Veal Broth

HIGH MEAT DINNERS

Beef with Vegetables
Chicken with Vegetables
Ham with Vegetables
Turkey with Vegetables
Veal with Vegetables

BREAKFASTS, DINNERS, AND SOUPS

Cereal, Egg Yolks, and Bacon
Chicken Soup
Oatmeal with Apples and Bananas
Rice Cereal with Apples and Bananas
Vegetables and Bacon
Vegetables and Beef
Vegetables and Ham with Bacon
Vegetables and Lamb

VEGETABLES

Beets
Carrots
Creamed Corn
Creamed Peas
Green Beans
Mixed Vegetables
Squash
Sweet Potatoes

DESSERTS

Custard Pudding
Fruit Dessert
Pineapple Orange Dessert
Tutti Frutti

Milk-Free Junior Foods

FRUITS
Apples and Cranberries
with Tapioca
Apples and Pears
Applesauce
Applesauce and Apricots
Apricots with Tapioca
Bananas and Pineapple
with Tapioca
Peaches
Pears
Pears and Pineapple

MEATS
Beef and Beef Broth
Chicken and Chicken
Broth
Lamb and Lamb Broth
Veal and Veal Broth

HIGH MEAT DINNERS
Beef with Vegetables
and Cereal
Chicken with Vegetables
Ham with Vegetables

BREAKFASTS, DINNERS,
AND SOUPS
Egg Noodles and Beef
Macaroni, Tomatoes,
Beef, and Bacon
Vegetables and Bacon
Vegetables and Beef
Vegetables, Dumplings,
Beef, and Bacon

VEGETABLES
Carrots
Green Beans
Mixed Vegetables
Sweet Potatoes

DESSERTS
Apple Pie
Banana Pie
Fruit Dessert
Peach Pie
Pineapple Orange
Dessert

Milk-Free Instant Cereals

Barley
Mixed

Oatmeal
Rice

Milk-Free Strained Foods

FRUITS
Apples and Cranberries
Apples and Pears

JUICES
Apple
Apple-Apricot

FRUITS
Applesauce
Applesauce and Apricots
Apricots with Tapioca
Bananas and Pineapple
Bananas with Tapioca
Peaches
Pears
Pears and Pineapple
Plums with Tapioca
Prunes with Tapioca

MEATS AND EGG YOLKS
Beef and Beef Broth
Chicken and Chicken
    Broth
Egg Yolks
Ham and Ham Broth
Lamb and Lamb Broth
Liver and Liver Broth
Pork and Pork Broth
Turkey and Turkey
    Broth
Veal and Veal Broth

HIGH MEAT DINNERS
Beef with Vegetables
Chicken with Vegetables
Ham with Vegetables
Veal with Vegetables

DESSERTS
Apple Pie
Banana Pie
Fruit Dessert
Peach Pie
Pineapple Orange
    Dessert

JUICES
Apple-Cherry
Apple-Grape
Apple-Pineapple
Apple-Prune
Mixed Fruit
Orange
Orange-Apple-Banana
Orange-Pineapple

BREAKFASTS, DINNERS,
    AND SOUPS
Beef and Egg Noodles
Mixed Cereal with
    Apples and Bananas
Oatmeal with Apples
    and Bananas
Rice Cereal with Apples
    and Bananas
Vegetables and Bacon
Vegetables and Beef
Vegetables and Ham
    with Bacon
Vegetables, Dumplings,
    Beef, and Bacon

VEGETABLES
Beets
Carrots
Green Beans
Mixed Vegetables
Squash
Sweet Pottaoes

Citrus-Fruit-Free Junior Foods

FRUITS

Apples and Cranberries
  with Tapioca
Apples and Pears
Applesauce
Applesauce and Apricots
Apricots with Tapioca
Peaches
Pears and Pineapple

BREAKFASTS, DINNERS,
  AND SOUPS

Cereal, Eggs and Bacon
Chicken Noodle Dinner
Egg Noodles and Beef
Macaroni, Tomatoes,
  Beef, and Bacon
Vegetables and Bacon
Vegetables and Beef
Vegetables and Ham
  with Bacon
Vegetables and Lamb
Vegetables, Dumplings,
  Beef, and Bacon
Vegetables, Egg
  Noodles, and Chicken
Vegetables, Egg
  Noodles, and Turkey

DESSERTS

Apple Pie
Custard Pudding
Peach Pie

MEATS

Beef and Beef Broth
Chicken and Chicken
  Broth
Chicken Sticks
Lamb and Lamb Broth
Meat Sticks
Veal and Veal Broth

HIGH MEAT DINNERS

Beef with Vegetables
  and Cereal
Chicken with Vegetables
Ham with Vegetables
Turkey with Vegetables
Veal with Vegetables

VEGETABLES

Carrots
Creamed Corn
Creamed Peas
Green Beans
Mixed Vegetables
Sweet Potatoes

Citrus-Fruit-Free Instant Cereals

Barley
High Protein
Mixed

Oatmeal
Rice

Citrus-Fruit-Free Strained Foods

FRUITS
Apples and Cranberries
Apples and Pears
Applesauce
Applesauce and Apricots
Apricots with Tapioca
Peaches
Pears
Pears and Pineapple
Plums with Tapioca
Prunes with Tapioca

MEATS AND EGG YOLKS
Beef and Beef Broth
Chicken and Chicken
    Broth
Egg Yolks
Ham and Ham Broth
Lamb and Lamb Broth
Liver and Liver Broth
Pork and Pork Broth
Turkey and Turkey
    Broth
Veal and Veal Broth

HIGH MEAT DINNERS
Beef with Vegetables
Chicken with Vegetables
Ham with Vegetables
Turkey with Vegetables
Veal with Vegetables

VEGETABLES
Beets
Carrots
Creamed Corn
Creamed Peas

Green Beans
Mixed Vegetables
Squash
Sweet Potatoes

JUICES
Apple
Apple-Apricot
Apple-Cherry
Apple-Grape
Apple-Pineapple
Apple-Prune

BREAKFASTS, DINNERS,
    AND SOUPS
Beef and Egg Noodles
Cereal, Egg Yolks, and
    Bacon
Chicken Noodle Dinner
Chicken Soup
Macaroni, Tomatoes,
    Beef, and Bacon
Mixed Cereal with
    Apples and Bananas
Oatmeal with Apples
    and Bananas
Vegetables and Bacon
Vegetables and Beef
Vegetables and Ham
    with Bacon
Vegetables and Lamb
Vegetables, Dumplings,
    Beef, and Bacon
Vegetables, Egg
    Noodles, and Chicken
Vegetables, Egg
    Noodles, and Turkey

DESSERTS
Apple Pie
Custard Pudding
Peach Pie

Egg-Free Junior Foods

FRUITS
Apples and Cranberries
  with Tapioca
Apples and Pears
Applesauce
Applesauce and Apricots
Apricots with Tapioca
Bananas and Pineapple
  with Tapioca
Cottage Cheese with
  Bananas
Peaches
Pears
Pears and Pineapple

MEATS
Beef and Beef Broth
Chicken and Chicken
  Broth
Chicken Sticks
Lamb and Lamb Broth
Meat Sticks
Veal and Veal Broth

HIGH MEAT DINNERS
Beef with Vegetables
  and Cereal
Chicken with Vegetables
Ham with Vegetables
Turkey with Vegetables
Veal with Vegetables

BREAKFASTS, DINNERS,
  AND SOUPS
Macaroni, Tomatoes,
  Beef, and Bacon
Vegetables and Bacon
Vegetables and Beef
Vegetables and Ham
  with Bacon
Vegetables and Lamb

VEGETABLES
Carrots
Creamed Corn
Creamed Peas
Green Beans
Mixed Vegetables
Sweet Potatoes

DESSERTS
Apple Pie
Banana Pie
Fruit Dessert
Peach Pie

INSTANT CEREALS
Barley
High Protein
Mixed
Oatmeal
Rice

Egg-Free Strained Foods

FRUITS
Apples and Cranberries
Apples and Pears
Applesauce
Applesauce and Apricots
Apricots with Tapioca
Bananas with Tapioca
Bananas with Pineapple
Cottage Cheese with Bananas
Peaches
Pears
Pears and Pineapple
Plums with Tapioca
Prunes with Tapioca

JUICES
Apple
Apple-Apricot
Apple-Cherry
Apple-Grape
Apple-Pineapple
Apple-Prune
Mixed Fruit
Orange
Orange-Apple-Banana
Orange-Pineapple

MEATS
Beef and Beef Broth
Chicken and Chicken Broth
Ham and Ham Broth
Lamb and Lamb Broth
Liver and Liver Broth
Pork and Pork Broth
Turkey and Turkey Broth
Veal and Veal Broth

HIGH MEAT DINNERS
Beef with Vegetables
Chicken with Vegetables
Ham with Vegetables
Turkey with Vegetables
Veal with Vegetables

BREAKFASTS, DINNERS, AND SOUPS
Chicken Soup
Macaroni, Tomatoes, Beef, and Bacon
Mixed Cereal with Apples and Bananas
Oatmeal with Apples and Bananas
Rice Cereal with Apples and Bananas
Vegetables and Bacon
Vegetables and Beef
Vegetables and Ham with Bacon
Vegetables and Lamb

VEGETABLES
Beets
Carrots
Creamed Corn
Creamed Peas
Green Beans
Mixed Vegetables
Squash
Sweet Potatoes

DESSERTS
Apple Pie
Banana Pie
Fruit Dessert
Peach Pie

Milk, Wheat, Egg, and Citrus-Fruit-Free Junior Foods

FRUITS
Apples and Cranberries
  with Tapioca
Apples and Pears
Applesauce
Applesauce and Apri-
  cots
Apricots with Tapioca
Peaches
Pears
Pears and Pineapple

HIGH MEAT DINNERS
Beef with Vegetables
  and Cereal
Chicken with Vegeta-
  bles
Ham with Vegetables
Veal with Vegetables

DINNERS
Vegetables and Bacon
Vegetables and Beef

MEATS
Beef and Beef Broth
Chicken and Chicken
  Broth
Lamb and Lamb Broth
Veal and Veal Broth

VEGETABLES
Carrots
Green Beans
Mixed Vegetables
Sweet Potatoes

Milk, Wheat, Egg, and Citrus-Fruit-Free Instant Cereals

Barley
Oatmeal

Rice

Milk, Wheat, Egg, and Citrus-Fruit-Free Strained Foods

FRUITS
Apples and Cranberries
Apples and Pears
Applesauce

Applesauce and Apri-
  cots
Apricots with Tapioca
Peaches

Pears
Pears and Pineapple
Plums with Tapioca
Prunes with Tapioca

JUICES
Apple
Apple-Apricot
Apple-Cherry
Apple-Grape
Apple-Pineapple
Apple-Prune

BREAKFASTS, DINNERS,
    AND SOUPS
Oatmeal with Apples
    and Bananas
Rice Cereal with Apples
    and Bananas
Vegetables and Bacon
Vegetables and Beef
Vegetables and Ham
    with Bacon

MEATS
Beef and Beef Broth
Chicken and Chicken
    Broth
Ham and Ham Broth
Lamb and Lamb Broth
Liver and Liver Broth
Pork and Pork Broth
Turkey and Turkey
    Broth
Veal and Veal Broth

HIGH MEAT DINNERS
Beef with Vegetables
Chicken with Vegetables
Ham with Vegetables
Veal with Vegetables

VEGETABLES
Beets
Carrots
Green Beans
Mixed Vegetables
Squash
Sweet Potatoes

Beech-Nut Baby Foods
The following allergy-free baby foods are manufactured by Beech-Nut.

Wheat-Free Strained Foods

PACKAGED CEREALS
Rice
Oatmeal
Honey Flavored Rice
Honey   Flavored   Oat-
    meal

HIGH MEAT DINNERS
Beef
Chicken
Ham
Turkey
Veal

JUICES
Apple
Apple-Cherry
Apple-Grape
Orange
Orange-Apple
Orange-Apricot
Orange-Banana
Orange-Pineapple
Orange-Prune
Mixed Fruit

MEATS AND EGG YOLKS
Beef
Chicken
Ham
Lamb
Pork
Turkey
Veal
Egg Yolks
Egg Yolks and Bacon

DESSERTS
Caramel Pudding
Peach Melba
Apple Betty
Chocolate Custard Pudding
Custard Pudding
Fruit Dessert with Tapioca
Orange Pineapple Dessert
Pineapple Dessert
Creamed Cottage Cheese
    with Pineapple Juice

VEGETABLES
Carrots
Carrots in Butter Sauce
Creamed Corn
Garden Vegetables
Green Beans
Peas
Peas in Butter Sauce
Squash
Squash in Butter Sauce
Sweet Potatoes
Sweet Potatoes in Butter Sauce

DINNERS AND SOUPS
Turkey Rice Dinner
Vegetable Soup
Vegetables and Bacon
Vegetables and Beef
Vegetables and Lamb
Vegetables and Liver
Oatmeal with Fruit

Egg-Free Strained Foods

PACKAGED CEREALS
Rice
Oatmeal
Mixed
Hi-Protein Cereal
Honey Flavored Rice
Honey Flavored Oat-
meal
Honey Flavored Mixed

JUICES
Apple
Apple-Cherry
Apple-Grape
Orange
Orange-Apple
Orange-Apricot
Orange-Banana
Orange-Pineapple
Orange-Prune
Mixed Fruit

MEAT AND EGG YOLKS
Beef
Chicken
Ham
Lamb
Pork
Turkey
Veal

HIGH MEAT DINNERS
Beef
Chicken
Ham
Turkey
Veal

VEGETABLES
Carrots
Carrots in Butter Sauce
Creamed Corn
Garden Vegetables
Green Beans
Green Beans in Butter
Sauce
Peas
Peas in Butter Sauce
Squash
Squash in Butter Sauce
Sweet Potatoes
Sweet Potatoes in But-
ter Sauce

DINNERS AND SOUPS
Chicken with Vegeta-
bles
Vegetable Soup
Turkey Rice Dinner
Vegetables and Bacon
Vegetables and Beef
Vegetables and Ham
Vegetables and Lamb
Vegetables and Liver
Oatmeal with Fruit
Mixed Cereal with Fruit

DESSERTS
Apple Betty
Fruit Dessert with Tapi-
oca
Creamed Cottage Cheese
with Pineapple Juice

Milk-Free Strained Foods

PACKAGED CEREALS
Oatmeal
Rice
Mixec
Hi-Protein
Honey Flavored Oat-
  meal
Honey Flavored Mixed
Honey Flavored Rice

FRUITS
Apple
Apple-Cherry
Apple-Grape
Orange
Orange-Apple
Orange-Apricot
Orange-Banana
Orange-Pineapple
Orange-Prune
Mixed Fruit

MEATS AND EGG YOLKS
Beef
Chicken
Ham
Lamb
Pork
Turkey
Veal
Egg Yolks
Egg Yolks and Bacon

HIGH MEAT DINNERS
Beef
Chicken
Ham
Turkey
Veal

VEGETABLES
Carrots
Garden Vegetables
Green Beans
Peas
Squash
Sweet Potatoes

DINNERS AND SOUPS
Chicken with Vegeta-
  bles
Vegetable Soup
Beef and Noodles
Chicken Noodle Dinner
Turkey Rice Dinner
Vegetables and Bacon
Vegetables and Beef
Vegetables and Lamb
Vegetables and Liver
Oatmeal with Fruit
Mixed Cereal with Fruit

DESSERTS
Fruit Dessert with Tapi-
  oca
Orange Pineapple Des-
  sert
Peach Melba

Citrus-Fruit-Free Strained Foods

PACKAGED CEREALS
Rice
Oatmeal
Mixed
Hi-Protein
Honey Flavored Rice
Honey Flavored Mixed
Honey Flavored Oatmeal

MEATS AND EGG YOLKS
Beef
Chicken
Ham
Lamb
Pork
Turkey
Veal
Egg Yolks
Egg Yolks and Bacon

HIGH MEAT DINNERS
Beef
Chicken
Ham
Turkey
Veal

VEGETABLES
Carrots
Carrots in Butter Sauce
Creamed Corn
Garden Vegetables
Green Beans
Green Beans in Butter Sauce
Peas

VEGETABLES
Peas in Butter Sauce
Squash
Squash in Butter Sauce
Sweet Potatoes
Sweet Potatoes in Butter Sauce

JUICES
Apple
Apple-Cherry
Apple-Grape

DINNERS AND SOUPS
Chicken with Vegetables
Vegetable Soup
Beef and Noodle Dinner
Macaroni, Tomato Sauce, Beef, and Bacon
Turkey Rice Dinner
Vegetables and Bacon
Vegetables and Beef
Vegetables and Ham
Vegetables and Lamb
Vegetables and Liver
Cereal, Egg Yolks, and Bacon

DESSERTS
Custard Pudding
Chocolate Custard Des-
sert
Pineapple Dessert
Creamed Cottage Cheese
with Pineapple Juice
Apple Betty
Caramel Pudding
Peach Melba

Wheat, Egg, Milk, and Citrus-Fruit-Free Foods

PACKAGED CEREALS
Rice
Honey Flavored Rice
Honey Flavored Mixed
Honey Flavored Oat-
meal

MEATS AND EGG YOLKS
Beef
Chicken
Ham
Lamb
Pork
Turkey

JUICES
Apple
Apple-Cherry
Apple-Grape

FRUITS
Applesauce
Applesauce and Cher-
ries
Applesauce and Rasp-
berries
Apples and Apricots
Apricots with Tapioca
Bananas with Tapioca
Bananas and Pineapple
with Tapioca
Peaches
Pears
Pears and Pineapple
Plums with Tapioca
Prunes with Tapioca

HIGH MEAT DINNERS
Beef
Chicken
Ham
Turkey
Veal

VEGETABLES
Carrots
Garden Vegetables
Green Beans
Peas
Squash
Sweet Potatoes

DINNERS AND SOUPS
Turkey Rice, Vegetable
  and Bacon
Vegetable Soup
Vegetables and Beef
Vegetables and Lamb
Vegetables and Liver

Wheat-Free Junior Foods

MEATS AND EGG YOLKS
Beef
Chicken
Chicken Sticks
Meat Sticks
Lamb
Pork
Turkey
Veal

HIGH MEAT DINNERS
Beef
Chicken
Ham
Turkey
Veal

DESSERTS
Peach Melba
Caramel Pudding
Apple Betty
Custard Pudding
Fruit Dessert with Tapi-
  oca
Tropical Fruit Dessert
Banana Dessert
Creamed Cottage Cheese
  with Pineapple

VEGETABLES
Carrots
Carrots in Butter Sauce
Peas in Butter Sauce
Green Beans
Squash
Squash in Butter Sauce
Sweet Potatoes
Sweet Potatoes in But-
  ter Sauce
Green Beans in Butter
  Sauce

DINNERS AND SOUPS
Vegetable Soup
Split Peas, Vegetable,
  and Ham
Turkey Rice Dinner
Vegetables and Bacon
Vegetables and Beef
Vegetables and Lamb
Vegetables and Liver

Egg-Free Junior Foods

MEATS AND EGG YOLKS
Beef
Chicken
Chicken Sticks
Meat Sticks
Lamb
Pork
Turkey
Veal

HIGH MEAT DINNERS
Beef
Chicken
Ham
Turkey
Veal

FRUITS
Applesauce
Applesauce and Cherries
Applesauce and Raspberries
Apples and Apricots
Peaches
Apples with Tapioca
Pears
Pears with Pineapple
Plums with Tapioca
Prunes with Tapioca
Banana and Pineapple with Tapioca

DINNERS AND SOUPS
Chicken with Vegetables
Vegetable Soup
Macaroni and Bacon with Vegetables
Macaroni and Beef with Vegetables
Spaghetti, Tomato Sauce, and Beef
Split Peas, Vegetables, and Ham
Turkey Rice Dinner
Vegetables and Bacon
Vegetables and Beef
Vegetables and Lamb
Vegetables and Liver

DESSERTS
Banana Dessert
Fruit Dessert with Tapioca
Tropical Fruit Dessert
Creamed Cottage Cheese with Pineapple
Peach Melba

VEGETABLES
Carrots
Carrots in Butter Sauce
Peas in Butter Sauce
Green Beans
Green Beans in Butter Sauce
Squash
Squash in Butter Sauce
Sweet Potatoes

VEGETABLES
Sweet Potatoes in but-
ter Sauce

Milk-Free Junior Foods

MEAT AND EGG YOLKS
Beef
Chicken
Lamb
Pork
Turkey
Veal

HIGH MEAT DINNERS
Beef
Chicken
Ham
Turkey
Veal

VEGETABLES
Carrots
Green Beans
Squash
Sweet Potatoes

DINNERS AND SOUPS
Chicken with Vegeta-
bles
Vegetable Soup
Beef and Noodles
Chicken Noodle Dinner
Macaroni and Beef with
Vegetables
Turkey Rice Dinner
Vegetables and Beef
Vegetables and Lamb
Vegetables and Liver

DESSERTS
Banana Dessert
Fruit Dessert with Tapi-
oca
Tropical Fruit Dessert
Peach Melba

Citrus-Fruit-Free Junior Foods

MEAT AND EGG YOLKS
Beef
Chicken
Chicken Sticks
Meat Sticks
Lamb
Turkey
Pork
Veal

HIGH MEAT DINNERS
Beef
Chicken
Ham

Turkey
Veal

VEGETABLES
Carrots
Carrots in Butter Sauce
Green Beans
Squash
Squash in Butter Sauce
Sweet Potatoes
Sweet Potatoes in But-
ter Sauce
Green Beans in Butter
Sauce

Peas
Peas in Butter Sauce

DINNERS AND SOUPS
Chicken with Vegetables
Cereal, Egg Yolks, and Bacon
Vegetable Soup
Beef and Noodles
Chicken and Noodles
Lamb and Noodles
MEATS AND EGG YOLKS
Macaroni and Bacon with Vegetables
Spaghetti, Tomato Sauce, and Beef
Split Peas, Vegetables, and Ham
Turkey Rice Dinner
Vegetables and Bacon
Vegetables and Beef
Vegetables and Lamb
Vegetables and Liver

DESSERTS
Custard Pudding
Creamed Cottage Cheese with Pineapple Juice
Apple Betty
Caramel Pudding
Peach Melba

FRUITS
Applesauce
Applesauce and Cherries
Applesauce and Raspberries
Apples and Apricots
Apricots with Tapioca
Peaches
Pears
Pears and Pineapple
Plums with Tapioca
Prunes with Tapioca

Wheat, Egg, Milk, and Citrus-Fruit-Free Junior Foods

MEATS AND EGG YOLKS
Beef
Chicken
Lamb
Pork
Turkey
Veal

HIGH MEAT DINNERS
Beef
Chicken

Ham
Turkey
Veal

VEGETABLES
Carrots
Green Beans
Squash
Sweet Potatoes

DINNERS AND SOUPS
Vegetable Soup
Turkey Rice Dinner

Vegetables and Beef
Vegetables and Lamb
Vegetables and Liver

Glossary

ADDITIVE. A drug which gives color or flavor to a preserved food.

ADRENAL GLANDS. Two glands in the upper posterior part of the abdomen which produce and secrete vital hormones. They have a *cortex,* which is the outer portion of the gland and is responsible for the production of cortisone, and a *medulla,* which is the central portion of the gland and is responsible for the production and secretion of adrenalin.

ADRENALIN (epinephrine). One of the hormones secreted by the adrenal glands.

ADRENERGIC. Referring to an adrenalin-like action.

ADRENOCORTICOTROPIC HORMONE (ACTH). The glandular secretion of the anterior portion of the pituitary gland in the base of the brain. This hormone influences the function of the adrenal and other glands of the body.

AEROSOL. A compressed gas containing particles of a substance to be used in the treatment of a patient. The medication is administered by releasing the compressed gas.

ALLERGEN. A substance that causes the formation of harmful antibodies leading to hypersensitivity and allergy.

ALLERGIC RHINITIS. An inflammation of the membranes of the nasal passages caused by an allergy such as hayfever.

ALLERGY. A sensitivity to some normally harmless substances, i.e., a pollen grain or milk.

ALTERNARIA. A fungus or mold which causes a form of hayfever.

ALVEOLI. An air cell of the lungs formed by the terminal dilation of tiny air passageways.

AMINO ACIDS. A large group of organic compounds, many of which are necessary for the maintenance of life. They represent an end product of protein metabolism.

AMINOPHYLLINE. A drug used to enlarge the blood vessels, lower the blood pressure, relieve asthmatic attacks, and stimulate urination.

ANAPHYLACTIC SHOCK. Shock produced by injecting a medication or substance to which the patient is allergic.

ANGIOEDEMA. Large hives.

ANTIBODY. The guard or defense agent produced by the body against an invading antigen.

ANTIGEN. A substance which enables a child to produce antibodies against it, i.e., a microbe or a virus.

ANTIHISTAMINE. A medication which counteracts an allergic reaction.

ANTIPRURITIC. A substance which relieves itching.

ATOPIC. Allergy-prone.

BLOCKING ANTIBODY. An antibody produced artificially by the injection of allergenic extracts.

BRONCHIOLES. The small bronchial tubes in the lungs which lead to the air cells.

BRONCHODILATOR. A medication which enlarges a spastic bronchial tube; often prescribed in acute asthma.

CAPILLARY. Small blood vessels.

COLLAGEN DISEASE. Any disease involving the connective tissues of the body.

CONJUNCTIVAL TEST. A test in which the substance suspected of being the cause of an allergy is dropped into the eye. Inflammation and redness shows a positive reaction.

CONTACT DERMATITIS. An inflammation of the skin due to contact with an irritant such as a chemical or a plant. Poison ivy, detergents, etc., may cause contact dermatitis.

CORTICOSTEROID. A chemical having the properties of the hormone secreted by the cortex or outer layer of the adrenal gland.

CORTISONE. A hormone secreted by the coretx of the adrenal gland.

CREAM. A salve made of a fat that can hold water and a medicine.

CROUP. An inflammation of the larynx accompanied by coughing, difficulty in breathing, fever, etc. It usually occurs in young children.

DANDER. Scales from the skin of hairy animals such as dogs, cats, horses, etc.

DERMOGRAPHIA OR "WRITING ON THE SKIN." A condition of the skin, wherein it becomes red and raised wherever it is irritated or scratched lightly.

ECZEMA. Any inflammatory disease of the skin.

EMPHYSEMA. A condition in which the air spaces in the lungs are enlarged. This makes breathing more difficult.

ENDOCRINE GLANDS. Glands which secrete their hormones into the bloodstream; such as the pituitary, thyroid, and adrenal glands. Also called *ductless glands*.

ENZYME. A substance manufactured by living tissue which stimulates specific chemical changes such as the breaking down of complex food proteins to reduce them to simpler structures which can be absorbed by the intestines.

EOSINOPHIL. A type of white blood cell which has a reddish color when stained and examined under a microscope. They increase in number when the patient has an allergic condition or when there is an invasion of the body by a parasite.

EPHEDRINE. A chemical with the same action as adrenalin.

EPINEPHRINE. The hormone secreted by the inner portion of the adrenal gland; also called adrenalin.

ERYTHEMA. A patch of redness on the skin.

FRONTAL SINUSES. The sinuses directly above the eyes.

FUNCTIONAL DISORDER. A disorder caused by uspet in function, not by actual organic disease processes.

FUNGUS. A form of plant life.

GAMMA GLOBULIN. A substance containing antibodies.

GLOBULINS OR IMMUNE-GLOBULINS. Special proteins found in the blood and some tissues. They are protective antibodies produced in response to an antigen. They react specifically to their antigen and neutralize it.

HAPTENS. Incomplete antigens.

HEREDITY. The passage of bodily characteristics or likelihood of disease from parent to offspring.

HISTAMINE. A product of protein metabolism which is important in causing allergy symptoms.

HISTORY. The record of symptoms and the sequence of events in an illness.

HIVES (urticaria). An allergic condition of the skin characterized by the formation of large blotches or welts which itch intensely.

HYPERSENSITIVITY. An abnormal bodily reaction to a substance normally found in the environment.

HYPOALLERGENIC. Least likely to evoke an allergic response.

HYPODERMIC. Beneath the skin.

HYPOSENSITIZATION. An effort to reduce hypersensitivity through a series of slowly increasing injections of the substance causing the allergy.

IMMUNE SERUM. A serum containing antibodies which can fight a specific disease.

IMMUNO-GLOBULIN E OR IgE. The specific globulin of allergy. Its previous name was skin-sensitizing antibody.

IMMUNIZATION. The process of making one immune to a disease.

INFLAMMATION. The reaction of tissues to injury, manifested by pain, heat, swelling, and redness.

INHALANT. An allergen that may be inhaled because it floats freely in the air.

LACTASE. An enzyme which digests the sugar found in milk.

LACTOSE. Milk sugar.

LEUKOCYTES. White blood cells.

LINIMENT. A salve made up of a powder and an oil.

LOBE. A rounded segment of an organ.

LOBULE. A small lobe.

LOTION. A powder suspended in water.

LYMPH. The fluid which is derived from connective tissue and tissue between organs. Lymph travels through lymph channels and lymph nodes (glands).

LYMPHOCYTE. A type of white blood cell having a single, rounded nucleus (cell center).

MANAGEMENT. The direction of the course of an allergic disorder until relieved or eliminated.

MAST CELL. Connective tissue cell which contains histamine.

MAXILLARY SINUSES. The sinuses located in the cheekbones.

MILLILITER (ml. or cc.). A unit of measurement (1/1000 of a liter).

MUCUS. A thick liquid secreted by mucous glands.

NEBULIZE. To convert a medication into a spray.

NEUTROPHIL. A white blood cell which fights infection.

OINTMENT. A salve consisting of a fat and a medicine dissolved in it.

PALPATION. The act of feeling an organ of the body in order to make a diagnosis.

PARANASAL SINUSES. The sinuses located around the nose.

PATCH TEST. A test to determine skin reactions to antigens. It is performed by applying the antigen to the skin, covering it with an adhesive patch, and inspecting it a day or two later for characteristic reactions.

PERENNIAL. Lasting throughout the year.

PHOTOSENSITIVITY. Sensitivity to light.

PHYSICAL EXAMINATION. The examination of the body by a physician, including investigation with such instruments as the stethoscope, blood pressure apparatus, fluoroscope, laboratory testing equipment, etc.

PHYSIOLOGY. The science dealing with the study of the function of tissues or organs.

PITUITARY GLAND. An important endocrine gland located at the base of the brain.

PNEUMOTHORAX. Air in the pleural cavity surrounding the lung.

POISON IVY. A vine which on contact can cause a skin inflammation.

POISON OAK. A plant which causes an inflammation similar to that of poison ivy.

POISON SUMAC. A shrub which causes a skin condition similar to that of poison ivy.

POLLEN. The male element of flowering plants.

POLLENOSIS. Sensitivity to pollen.

POLYP. A nonmalignant growth in a mucous membrane.

PRICKLY HEAT. A skin rash brought on by excessive heat and perspiration.

PROTEIN NITROGEN UNITS OR PNU. A unit of measurement used in skin testing and desensitizing solutions.

PROTOPLASM. The essential materials making up living cells.

PRURITIS. Itch.

PUBERTY. The period of life when the sex organs begin to mature.

PYLOROSPASM. Severe spasm of the sphincter muscle of the pylorus.

PYLORUS. The far end of the stomach just before the duodenum.

RAGWEED. A weed whose pollen causes hayfever.

SALINE SOLUTION. A solution containing nine grams of kitchen salt in one liter of water.

SATURATED. Having all the solids or gases which a solution can take dissolved in it.

SEBORRHEIC DERMATITIS. A skin disease due to oversecretion of the sebaceous glands.

SERUM. That part of the blood which remains liquid after it has clotted. (See immune serum and serum sickness.)

SERUM SICKNESS. Fever, hives, and enlargement of lymph glands occurring seven to ten days after receiving an antitoxin containing animal serum.

SHOCK. An upset caused by inadequate amounts of blood circulating in the bloodstream. It may be caused by many conditions, including allergy. (See anaphylactic shock.)

SHOCK ORGAN. The organ of the body in which the allergic reaction takes place and where the symptoms manifest themselves.

SINUSES. The hollow spaces in the bones surrounding the nose.

SINUSITIS. Inflammation of one of the sinuses.

SMALLPOX. A highly contagious disease with a characteristic skin eruption. It occurs in epidemic form and can be prevented by vaccination.

SPHENOID SINUSES. The sinuses behind and above the nose. It has an outlet which drains into the nasal cavity.

SPORE. The reproductive cell of a mold.

SPUTUM. Mucous material spit out of the mouth. It may arise from the nose, throat, windpipe, or lungs.

SQUAMOUS. Resembling the scales of a fish. Squamous cells line certain body surfaces.

STATUS ASTHMATICUS. An asthma which does not respond to classical medication.

STEROIDS. Drugs of hormone origin, especially those from the pituitary and adrenal glands.

STRESS REACTIONS. Abnormal condition or disorders caused by undue stress or the tensions of living.

SUBCUTANEOUS. Underneath the skin.

SULFONAMIDES. The sulfa drugs.

SUNSTROKE. Inability of the body to rid itself of excessive heat. Body temperatures may rise as high as 106° to 108°F.

SWEAT TEST. Examination of sweat for its chemical composition performed on infants in cases of suspected pancreatic fibrosis.

SYMPTOMATIC TREATMENT. Treatment which is directed toward relieving the patient's complaints rather than toward getting at the basic cause of the illness.

SYSTEM. A set of organs performing one main function, such as the respiratory system (breathing).

SYSTEMIC. Referring to a condition or disease involving the entire body, as opposed to a localized condition.

TARTRAZINE. An additive.

TEST. A procedure to aid in making a diagnosis. (See conjunctival test.)

THEOPHYLLINE. An asthma medication which relaxes the bronchial muscles and causes the excretion of large amounts of urine.

THYMUS GLAND. A gland composed of a special

type of lymphoid tissue, located beneath the breastbone. It shrinks and becomes inactive early in childhood.

THYROID GLAND. The endocrine gland in the front of the neck which controls body metabolism.

TONSILS. Lymph glands located in the mouth near the back of the tongue.

TONSILLECTOMY. Removal of the tonsils.

TOXIN. The poison manufactured by germs or other forms of animal or vegetable life.

TRACHEA. The windpipe.

TYMPANIC MEMBRANE. The eardrum.

VACCINATION. The giving of a vaccine to prevent the onset of a disease.

WET DRESSING. A watery solution used to provide moisture to the skin.

Index

195

About the Author
EMILE SOMEKH, M.D.

Fellow of the American Association for Clinical Immunology and Allergy

Fellow of the Royal Society of Health
London, England

Diplomate in Pediatrics
Rome University, Italy

Teaching Assistant in Pediatric Allergy
St. Vincent's Hospital, New York

Former Teaching Assistant in Pediatric Allergy
New York University and North Shore Hospital, New York

Former Fellow of the National Jewish Institute for Asthmatic Children, Denver